Public Health: Practices, Methods and Policies (Edited Series)

Joav Merrick (Series Editor)
Division for Intellectual and Developmental Disabilities, Ministry of Social Affairs and Social Services, Jerusalem, Israel

"Public Health" is a book series with publications from a multidisciplinary group of researchers, practitioners and clinicians for an international professional forum interested in the broad spectrum of public health issues.

About the Editor-in-Chief
Joav Merrick, MD, MMedSci, DMSc, born and educated in Denmark is Professor of Pediatrics affiliated with the Division of Pediatrics, Hadassah Hebrew University Medical Center, Mt Scopus Campus, Jerusalem, Israel, Kentucky Children's Hospital, University of Kentucky, Lexington, United States and Professor of Public Health at the Center for Healthy Development, School of Public Health, Georgia State University, Atlanta, United States, the former medical director of the Disability Administration, Ministry of Social Affairs and Social Services, Jerusalem and the founder and director of the National Institute of Child Health and Human Development in Israel. Email: jmerrick@zahav.net.il

nova
Medicine & Health
New York

Public Health: Practices, Methods and Policies (Edited Series)

Public Health: Implications of Health Behaviors and Diseases
Emmanuel O Keku, MD, MA, MSPH
Joav Merrick, MD, MMedSci, DMSc
(Editors)
2023. ISBN: 979-8-89113-083-8 (Hardcover)
2023. ISBN: 979-8-89113-232-0 (eBook)

Positive Youth Development: The Tin Ka Ping P.A.T.H.S. Project in Mainland China
Daniel T.L. Shek, PhD, FHKPS, BBS, SBS, (Editor)
Moon YM Law, RSW, MSW, (Editor)
Xiaoqin Zhu, (Editor)
Joav Merrick, MD, MMedSci, DMSc (Editor)
2022. ISBN: 979-8-88697-282-5 (Softcover)
2022. ISBN: 979-8-88697-324-2 (eBook)

Public Health: Recent International Research
Joav Merrick, MD, MMedSci, DMSc (Editor), Mohammed Morad, MD (Editor)
2022. ISBN: 978-1-68507-491-3 (Hardcover)
2022. ISBN: 978-1-68507-638-2 (eBook)

Environmental Justice and the Intersection of Poverty, Racism and Child Health Disparities
I. Leslie Rubin, MD (Editor), Joav Merrick, MD, MMedSci, DMSc (Editor)
2022. ISBN: 978-1-68507-489-0 (Hardcover)
2022. ISBN: 978-1-68507-640-5 (eBook)

Science, Culture, and Politics: Despair and Hope in the Time of a Pandemic
Consolato M. Sergi, MD (Author)
2021. ISBN: 978-1-53619-816-4 (Hardcover)
2021. ISBN: 978-1-68507-161-5 (eBook)

More information about this series can be found at
https://novapublishers.com/product-category/series/public-health-practices-methods-and-policies/

Emmanuel O Keku
and Joav Merrick
Editors

Public Health

Implications of Health Behaviors and Diseases

nova
Medicine & Health
New York

DOI: https://doi.org/10.52305/GRGM2881

NOTICE TO THE READER

Library of Congress Cataloging-in-Publication Data

Names: Keku, Emmanuel O., editor. | Merrick, Joav, 1950- editor.
Title: Public health: implications of health behaviors and diseases / Emmanuel O. Keku, editor, Professor and Track Director, MD/MPH Program, Department of Public Health and Preventive Medicine, School of Medicine, St. George's University, St. George, Grenada, West Indies, Joav Merrick, MD, MMedSci, DMSc, editor, Medical Director, Health Services, Division for Intellectual and Developmental Disabilities, Ministry of Social Affairs and Social Services, Jerusalem, Israel, Division of Adolescent Medicine, KY Children's Hospital, Department of Pediatrics, Lexington, Kentucky, USA, National Institute of Child Health and Human Development, Jerusalem, Israel, Division of Pediatrics, Hadassah Hebrew University Medical Centers, Mt. Scopus Campus, Jerusalem, Israel, School of Public Health, Georgia State University, Atlanta, Georgia, USA.
Description: New York : Nova Science Publishers, [2023] | Series: Public health: practices, methods and policies | Includes bibliographical references and index. |
Identifiers: LCCN 2023041593 (print) | LCCN 2023041594 (ebook) | ISBN 9798891130838 (hardcover) | ISBN 9798891132320 (adobe pdf)
Subjects: LCSH: Health behavior. | Health status indicators. | Public health. | Medicine, Preventive.
Classification: LCC RA776.9 .P83 2023 (print) | LCC RA776.9 (ebook) | DDC 362.1--dc23/eng/20230925
LC record available at https://lccn.loc.gov/2023041593
LC ebook record available at https://lccn.loc.gov/2023041594

Published by Nova Science Publishers, Inc. † New York

Contents

Section one: Introduction

Chapter 1

Public health implications of health behaviors and diseases

Emmanuel O Keku[1], MD, MA, MSPH
Abidemi Fasanmi[1], MD, MPH, PhD
Anthony La[1], BA
and Joav Merrick[2-5], MD, MMedSci, DMSc
[1]Department of Public Health and Preventive Medicine, St George's University, School of Medicine, St George, Grenada, West Indies
[2]National Institute of Child Health and Human Development, Jerusalem, Israel
[3]Department of Pediatrics, Mt Scopus Campus, Hadassah Medical Center and Faculty of Medicine, Hebrew University of Jerusalem, Jerusalem, Israel
[4]Kentucky Children's Hospital, University of Kentucky, Lexington, Kentucky, United States of America
[5]Center for Healthy Development, School of Public Health, Georgia State University, Atlanta, Georgia, United States of America

Introduction

A central objective of public health practice and policy development is to influence health behavior change. During the pre-COVID-19 era, this core objective of public health was observed in the significant increase of global support for the public health field with increasing attention to preventing exposures to unhealthy behaviors, and risk factors and encouraging healthy lifestyle practices through behavioral modifications. The public health practitioners were excited about the positive outcomes of these interventions at private, public, and professional levels. However, bridging the disparities gap is still a problem. Globally, there are major health disparities issues

In: Public Health
Editors: Emmanuel O Keku and Joav Merrick
ISBN: 979-8-89113-083-8

concerning healthcare, vaccination, prevention of diseases, and treatment of diseases. The disparity gap is also increasing between racial groups and countries. The present COVID-19 era significantly exposed the complexities of these disparities within healthcare practices such as access to care, vaccination, and treatments for COVID-19 both within and across countries.

Public health practitioners are obligated to seek ways to improve access to healthcare services and decrease health disparities. It is important to emphasize that the issues of accessibility to healthcare and health disparities are of major concern to public health practitioners globally. Some way this could be achieved is to improve health literacy, especially when it comes to improving vaccination rates globally. Within the context of improving health literacy, we see a significant need for supporting roles for public health researchers, behavioral scientists, health educators, health promoters, health communicators, epidemiologists, environmentalists, and governments in policy development, implementation and monitoring, and evaluation.

Influence behavior change

To decrease morbidity and mortality of diseases within populations, public health practitioners need to influence behavior change at multiple levels: the individual, community, and institutions. For an individual, knowledge, and understanding of how health behaviors and exposures to risk factors for disease development are essential and linked to positive behavior change and healthy choices. Similarly, communities and institutional changes aimed at social, economic, and environmental changes are needed to eliminate social and structural barriers that limit or prevent access to health literacy, and healthcare services, hinder positive behavior choices and increase healthcare costs, thereby, reducing the quality of life.

Though chronic diseases dominate the leading causes of death globally, we are beginning to see emerging infectious diseases such as COVID-19 and Ebola. The systematic methods we develop to control both chronic and infectious diseases in the populations should be focused and include addressing issues such as access to healthcare and health disparities which are often overlooked. In this COVID-19 era, an ongoing public health assessment, interventions, and monitoring of health behaviors is key to improving holistic public health activities. This effort must encompass preventive and treatment interventions at public, private, and governmental levels. Although the effects are not always initially apparent, implementing a preventive approach proves to be an effective way of saving future implied health care costs of those who would have accrued a condition. It is important to understand that an overall healthier community would naturally lead to decreased burden on healthcare infrastructures both financially and operationally.

Prevention

Preventive approaches such as education or increased screening can theoretically decrease incidences of chronic diseases that require expensive long-term management of care. The government of each country must also determine and implement health policies that promote prevention and provide healthcare services in a sustainable and cost-efficient manner. It is essential to emphasize that governmental health policies that encourage ongoing cost-benefit analyses or effectiveness of resource allocations will improve the health outcomes of their populations and control both chronic and emerging infectious diseases within their countries. Middle- and low-income countries often have a difficult decision to make when it comes to the allocation of their healthcare resources due to limited healthcare resources, and these countries tend to allocate a significant amount of healthcare resources to infectious disease control than chronic diseases. This decision is associated with the urgency to mitigate infectious disease outbreaks and their immediate outcome, which is more devastating than that of chronic diseases, even though, chronic diseases are more costly to treat and often lead to poor quality of life. It is, therefore, pertinent that public health practitioners encourage governments to allocate healthcare resources equitably to both infectious and chronic diseases.

Conclusion

The pre-Covid 19 era observed significant global support for the public health field with increasing attention to preventing exposures to unhealthy behaviors, and risk factors and encouraging healthy lifestyle practices through behavioral modifications. Ironically, COVID-19 pandemic show that more is needed to eliminate the social and structural barriers that limit or prevent access to health literacy, and healthcare services, hinder positive behavior choices and increase healthcare costs, thereby, reducing the quality of life. The global pandemic, consequently, exposed the need for transformational and sustainable health policies geared towards effective ways of saving future implied health care costs due to preventable communicable and/or noncommunicable diseases. It furthermore confirmed the need for a concerted effort by the public, private, and government on addressing issues such as access to healthcare and health disparities which are often overlooked and facilitating communities and institutional changes aimed at promoting social, economic, and environmental health.

Section two: Health behaviors and disease

Chapter 2

Particulate matter and infant mortality: A narrative review

Jenniffer T Graffam[1], MD, MPH
Anthony La[1], BA
Ifeoluwa Afon[1], BS
Uyioghosa Idahor[1], BS
Tolulope Oladimeji[2], MD, MPH
Kerry Mitchell[1], PhD
and Emmanuel O Keku[1], MD, MA, MSPH
[1]Department of Public Health and Preventive Medicine, St George's University, School of Medicine, St George, Grenada, West Indies
[2]Department of Pathophysiology, St George's University, School of Medicine, St George, Grenada, West Indies

Abstract

Air pollution, specifically particulate matter (PM), is a current public health concern due to its significant impact on human health. Two kinds of particulate matter are present in the atmosphere: PM_{10} and $PM_{2.5}$. The most health damaging is $PM_{2.5}$ since it can penetrate the lung barrier and enter the blood system causing cardiovascular and respiratory diseases as well as cancers if there is chronic exposure. Diverse studies have researched the effects of PM and its association with infant mortality. The purpose of this narrative review is to evaluate the literature concerning PM and infant mortality to establish the need for stricter environmental policies in countries where PM concentration exceeds the World Health Organization (WHO) guidelines. A collection of articles between 2008 and 2020 concerning PM and infant mortality were

In: Public Health
Editors: Emmanuel O Keku and Joav Merrick
ISBN: 979-8-89113-083-8

selected using databases including Google Scholar, Medline, PubMed, and ScienceDirect, in addition to public databases such as the WHO and the United States Environmental Protection Agency. Articles that considered air pollutants other than PM were excluded and the analysis of the data was done to propose future recommendations. Different studies conclude that $PM_{2.5}$ is associated with infant mortality on a global scale. In fact, anthropogenic $PM_{2.5}$ is significantly more detrimental than natural $PM_{2.5}$, so it is recommended that the WHO lowers the limit of $PM_{2.5}$ in the air from 10 μg m^{-3}.

Keywords: particulate matter, infant mortality, $PM_{2.5}$ concentration, air pollutants

Introduction

Air pollution is considered a worldwide threat for human health and a public health concern. Multiple studies have revealed robust evidence about the adverse health effects such as premature mortality. These effects include but are not limited to respiratory and cardiovascular diseases due to short term and long-term exposure to air pollution. According to the World Health Organization (WHO), nine out of 10 people are exposed to air quality that exceeds the limit of air pollutants allowed by WHO guidelines (1). In fact, in a recent study, air pollution was estimated to cause 8.8 million premature deaths in 2015. One dangerous element of air pollution is particulate matter (PM), which is considered to be the deadliest form due to its microscopic size and ability to enter the bloodstream (2).

PM is a component of atmospheric air; it is a mixture of solid and liquid particles that when present, enters the respiratory system along with the oxygen needed to breathe. The major components of PM are sulfate, nitrates, ammonia, sodium chloride, black carbon, mineral dust, and water (1). Particulate matter includes PM_{10} that consists of inhalable particles that are 10 micrometers in diameter and $PM_{2.5}$, which are particles with a diameter of 2.5 or smaller (3).

The most health damaging is $PM_{2.5}$ which is small enough to enter the lungs and oxidize the pneumocytes, increasing the risk of cancer. Additionally, this reaction causes inflammation, irritation, and blocked airflow, leading to cardiovascular and respiratory diseases (1). $PM_{2.5}$ is also found in carbon-based compounds which creates a challenge for areas of the world where carbon is present in households and is still a major source of energy environmentally. Consequences of early and daily exposure to $PM_{2.5}$ include serious health threats. Both in utero and during the first year of life, infants breathe $PM_{2.5}$ microscopic particulars which attack their vulnerable immune system and adversely affect the development of increasing infant morbidity and mortality.

According to the Center for Disease Control (4) infant mortality is defined as the death of an infant before his/her first birthday and the rate is calculated by the number of dead infants over 1,000 live births (4). It is estimated that 2.5 million children die annually in the first 28 days of life. Concurrently, the WHO estimates that globally, over 4.2 million deaths are due to ambient air pollution specially $PM_{2.5}$.

A strong association between PM and infant mortality has been discussed in the literature, this association is more evident in developing countries where levels of PM tend to be higher, yet evidence has also been found in countries such as Canada and the United States (5). Maternal exposure to $PM_{2.5}$ has been associated with a higher risk of preterm birth (< 37 weeks). Preterm birth generally consists of many risk factors such as neurological and physical developmental disabilities. Coupled with $PM_{2.5}$ exposure, these developmental risks are greater (6). Yorifuji et al. (7) also comments that $PM_{2.5}$ was associated with increased risk of infant and post-neonatal mortality, especially for mortality related to respiratory causes (7).

This paper aims to consolidate some of the literature about the association between infant mortality and particulate matter, and further analyze the relevance of this correlation. In addition, this narrative review intends to evaluate the need for more strict environmental policies among developing countries and/or countries where PM concentration exceeds the WHO guidelines. The goal is then to achieve, through this analysis, the reassessment of the WHO guidelines in order to reduce the prevalence of the problem, educate communities, and focus the issue of PM and infant mortality as a main public concern threatening infantile health.

Methods

The search engines Google Scholar and PubMed, and the databases Medline and ScienceDirect were used to collect relevant literature. The key words used were: Particulate matter and infant mortality as major concepts as well as association between air pollution and infant mortality. The time period considered was from 2008 to 2020. In addition, a search in the websites of the

World Health Organization (WHO) and United States Environmental Protection Agency (EPA) were considered as sources for statistical and factual information.

Articles that specifically explored the role of PM_{10} and $PM_{2.5}$ on infant health were selected. Inclusion criteria consisted of studies done between 2008-2020 particularly in developing or developed countries. Comparatively, studies done with a global approach were also selected; articles must include PM as the main air pollutant being studied. Thus, any study that did not specifically address infantile health and PM, addressed other components of air pollution other than PM, or only discussed PM effects on adults was excluded.

Analysis

The results given by the electronic search were read and verified for relevance. Figure 1 below is a diagram of the literature search showing the articles were divided into those whose research was done at a global scale and those done at a country/area specific level. Based on data collected, conclusions about the effect of particulate matter, specifically $PM_{2.5}$, and infantile mortality were drawn to give a recommendation and guidelines for future research.

Results

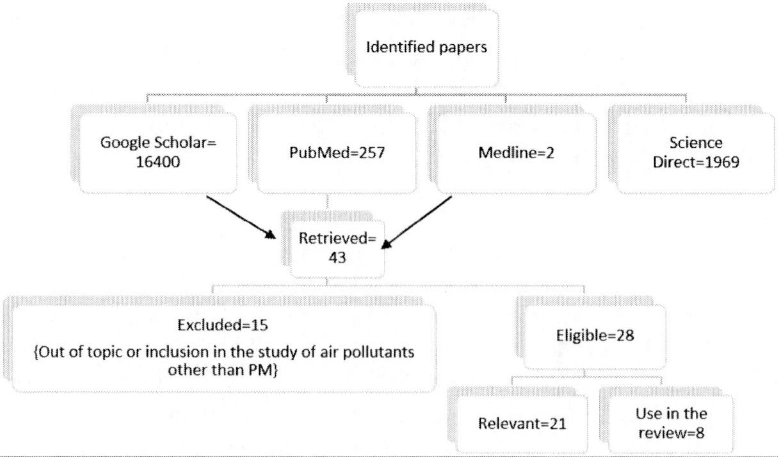

Figure 1. Diagram of literature search.

Discussion

Infant mortality has a higher prevalence in preterm births which are associated with an increased risk of death or complications due to physical or neurological causes; these causes occur at higher propensity compared with full term births. $PM_{2.5}$ exposure and its correlation with preterm births has been largely studied in Canada, China, and the United States (6). Nonetheless, the first study to analyze and calculate the implications of the $PM_{2.5}$ exposure with preterm births on a global scale was not published until 2017. In this study Malley et al. (6) presents data from 183 countries and integrates studies done in Latin America, Asia, Africa, North America and Europe.

On a global scale, the $PM_{2.5}$ association with preterm birth was around 2.7 million at a concentration of 10 $\mu g\ m^{-3}$ and 3.4 million with a concentration of 4.3 $\mu g\ m^{-3}$. South and East Asia, North and West sub-Saharan Africa had the largest contribution to the global total and the largest number of preterm births (6).

According to Malley (6), independently of the concentration, South and East Asia were the biggest contributors of preterm births associated with $PM_{2.5}$. Both areas contribute to 75% (10 $\mu g\ m^{-3}$) and 65% (4.3 $\mu g\ m^{-3}$) respectively (6). Specifically, the Eastern Asian country China held a significant portion of this data. Although China's mortality rate was low, a large number of live births and population-weighted $PM_{2.5}$ concentration was above the 98th percentile placing the country as the second largest contributor to infant mortality due to PM pollution. Population-weighted is a population average for urban settings in a country and it refers to the mean annual concentration of fine suspended particles less than 2.5 microns in diameter according to the WHO (1). Moreover, the African region contributed to more than 5% of the global data regardless of the PM concentration. Owili et al. (8) argues that $PM_{2.5}$ in Western and Central Africa increased infant mortality by 2% and 19% respectively, and anthropogenic $PM_{2.5}$ overall increased infant mortality in Africa by 5 to 10% (8).

The number of preterm births associated with $PM_{2.5}$ globally was not just dominated by countries with a high population-weighted average, but also by countries with a moderately low average. Countries such as Indonesia, Brazil, the United States and Uganda were part of the top 10% based on their large number of preterm births and air pollution data (6).

Malley et al. (6) results support the need to reduce $PM_{2.5}$ anthropogenic pollutants concentration. For example, the main contributing areas of South and East Asia between 81% to 85% of $PM_{2.5}$ were anthropogenic and as well as 21% in other areas such as West sub-Saharan Africa, North Africa and the Middle East. Malley (6) states that globally, 2.7 million preterm births were associated only with anthropogenic production of $PM_{2.5}$: equivalent to 81% of the total number of preterm births.

In a different global analysis, Goyal, Karra and Canning (9) found similar results. In this study, data from half a million births from 69 different countries was analyzed between 1998 and 2004. In this analysis, the main points were to evaluate early exposure to $PM_{2.5}$ and infant mortality. Infant mortality was subdivided in two categories: neonatal mortality that occurs in the first 28 days of life and post-neonatal infant mortality that occurs between 28 days of life and end of first year of life. This analysis improves two previous studies done in Mexico City and Brazil where infant death before age five years and air pollution was studied and found a strong correlation between mortality and exposure to PM within a few days of death (9).

The mean exposure to overall $PM_{2.5}$ in the study was 24.43 10 μg m^{-3}; this is a concentration that exceeds by more than double the WHO recommendation of 10 μg m^{-3}, but the mean exposure to $PM_{2.5}$ without naturally generated dust and sea-salt was 13.55 μg m^{-3}. Areas of the world such as Nepal, India and sub-Saharan countries have high levels of pollution due to biomass burning (9).

Anthropogenic $PM_{2.5}$ was of particular importance in the latest study since the results show that there is not a strong correlation between early life exposure to natural (dust and sea-salt) $PM_{2.5}$ and infant mortality. However, there is a strong correlation suggested by the author, between $PM_{2.5}$ from carbonaceous sources and infant mortality, especially neonatal mortality. Figure 2 shows that the composition and the levels of toxicity of PM are significant. This indicates that pollution generated by human activity has the highest burden in children's health and development.

A vast number of similar results have been found in other studies. For example, a study conducted in the United States in 2008, found a strong correlation between PM in the air and post neonatal mortality; particularly deaths due to respiratory causes (3). A different study from 2011 in Seoul Korea evaluated 359,459 subjects and found a significant relationship between gestational PM exposure and infant mortality due to all causes; there was a stronger correlation between particulate matter exposure and respiratory causes of death. The study goes further to argue that the prenatal exposure to $PM_{2.5}$ alters the fetus' health through inflammation, altering blood coagulation and reduces heart rate variability (10).

Furthermore, in a more recent study researched in Africa, it was found that 9.2% of infant deaths were associated with $PM_{2.5}$ exposure in the first 12 months of life (11). In fact, 22% of infant deaths were due to exposure to $PM_{2.5}$ concentrations above the minimum recommended levels by the WHO. Heft-Neal et al. (11) mention that they estimate a positive association between

$PM_{2.5}$ exposure and mortality at levels below the WHO recommended guidelines of 10 μg m^{-3} annual average (1) this is described in Figure 3.

Strengths and limitations

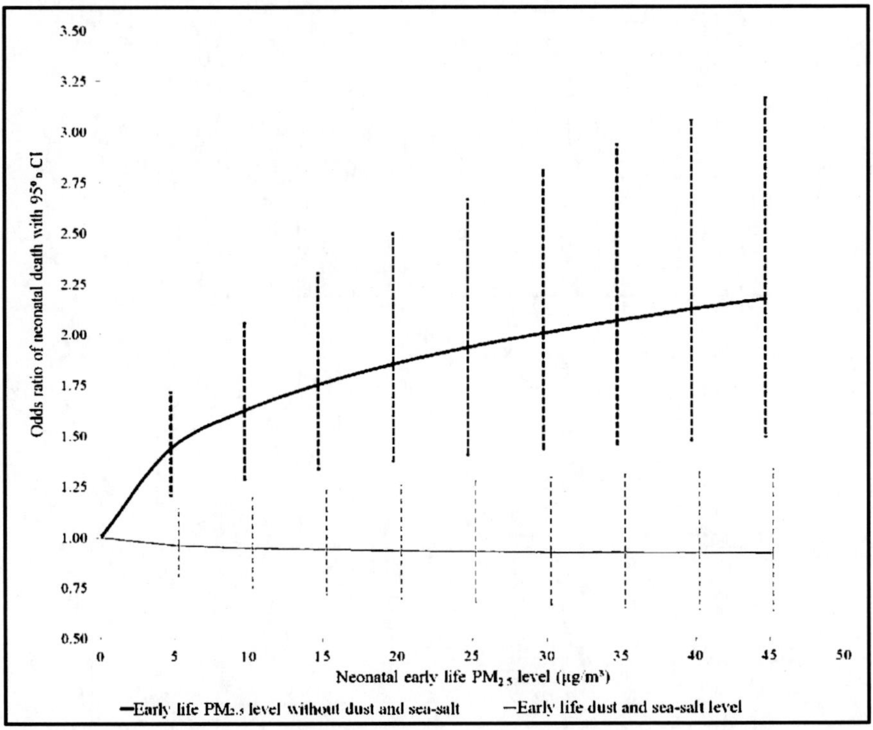

Figure 2. Odds ratio and corresponding 95% confidence intervals of neonatal death due to exposure to anthropogenic $PM_{2.5}$ levels and exposure to dust and sea-salt $PM_{2.5}$ (9).

Table 1. Studies assessing the relationship between particulate matter and infant mortality

Study	Study Location and Analyzed period	Methodology	Results	Interpretation
Chen X, et al. (2017)	116 Cities in China (2006-2012)	Survey data of respiratory disease mortality.	The effect of air pollutants has an impact on public health since emissions of air pollutants lead to an increase of 0.035 and 0.03 per ten thousand persons in local mortalities due to respiratory causes.	The article focused on air pollution and PM as a public health threat. The information is of use to support the initial hypothesis.
Goyal N. & Canning D (2019)	43 low- and middle-income countries (1998-2014)	Data from more than 500.000 births from 69 Demographic and Health Surveys.	Weak association between overall $PM_{2.5}$ level and infant mortality (OR: 1,00, 95% CI: 0.99,1,00). However, there is a strong association between exposure to $PM_{2.5}$ without dust and sea-salt and neonatal mortality. The odds of neonatal mortality increase with increased exposure to early life $PM_{2.5}$ without dust and sea-salt (OR 1.22; 95% CI: 1.11, 1.35). The data also indicates that doubling the level of $PM_{2.5}$ is associated with 14.9% increase in the odds of neonatal mortality. Deaths before the age of 1 are also robust (OR: 1.13; 95% CI: 1.04, 1.23), here, a doubling level of $PM_{2.5}$ without dust or sea salt increases odds of mortality by 8.8%.	The study acknowledges the possibility of residual confounding from omitted variables related to $PM_{2.5}$ exposure and child mortality. However, it concludes that their data is strong enough to suggest that children exposed to $PM_{2.5}$ without dust and sea salt have significantly higher odds of neonatal mortality (even at levels well below the WHO-recommended guideline).

Study	Study Location and Analyzed period	Methodology	Results	Interpretation
Heft-Neal, et. al. (2018)	30 countries from sub-Saharan Africa (2001-2015)	990,696 births using 65 Demographic and Health Surveys.	Modeling the effects of $PM_{2.5}$ exposure on infant mortality using fixed-effect regression analysis found a strong and linear correlation with $PM_{2.5}$ and infant death. A 10 μg m^{-3} increase in $PM_{2.5}$ exposure in the first 12 months of life is associated with a 9.2% increase in infant mortality ($P < 0.01$). No findings about differences between exposure before and after birth. An exposure to $PM_{2.5}$ higher than 2 was associated with 449,000 (95%; CI 194,000-709,000) additional infant deaths in 2015 alone. Similar associations were found in a dataset restricted to West Africa versus the rest of Africa and there was no evidence that wealth was a protective factor.	The authors estimated that reducing $PM_{2.5}$ concentrations uniformly by 5 μg m^{-3} at all locations could achieve a reduction in infant mortality of 4.6% and avoid 40,000 (95%; CI: 20,000-70,000) deaths in 2015 alone. They also found a strong association between in utero $PM_{2.5}$ exposure and neonatal deaths, and negative association with birth weight, post birth stunting and diarrhea. These findings argue in favor of changing the current guidelines.
Malley C, et al. (2017)	183 countries in 2010	The number of live births and preterm births estimated by a study in 2012 was used for the 183 countries. The data was collected from National registries, national surveys, and peer-reviewed literature.	In 2010 the number of preterm births related to only anthropogenic $PM_{2.5}$ was 2.7 million at a concentration of 10 μg m^3. There were additional 3.4 million related cases at concentrations of 4.3 μg m^3. Globally 18% of all preterm births were associated with a $PM_{2.5}$ concentration of 10 μg m^{-3}. The countries with the largest percentages (above the 90th percentile) were South and East Asia, North/middle and east Africa, and West sub-Sahara	The study analysis also emphasizes the contribution of $PM_{2.5}$ effects in utero which increases postnatal mortality and lifetime morbidity. This information is of great importance since the negative correlation between PM and infantile health may start in the prenatal period, increasing the urgency for action.

Table 1. (Continued)

Study	Study Location and Analyzed period	Methodology	Results	Interpretation
Owili P, et al. (2017)	54 Countries in Africa are divided into 5 sub-geographical regions. (2000- 2015).	Total- population data were based on the de facto definition of population which included all counted residents regardless of legal status or citizenship.	Results show that $PM_{2.5}$ concentration and under-five mortality was significant in all the study's sub-regions ($p < 0.001$). The under-five children who had exposure to mixed particles for 12 months had an increase in incidence of death 1.01 (95%; CI: 1.01-1.02) and as the year progressed the incidence increased by 34%. Biomass $PM_{2.5}$ had a positive association with under-five death ($B = 0.02$, $p < 0.001$). Anthropogenic $PM_{2.5}$ increased the under-five mortality by 4% in East Africa and dust $PM_{2.5}$ increased the under-five mortality by 3% (North Africa), 1% (Western) and 10% (Central Africa).	Another example of a large study that found relevant data in different areas of Africa and in different socio- economic backgrounds. The impact of anthropogenic $PM_{2.5}$ is evident based on the results from the data collected.
Scheers H, et al. (2011)	Flanders-Belgium (1998-2006).	2,455 infants	During the period of study, PM concentration averaged 31.8 +/- 13.8 $\mu g\ m^{-3}$ and 321 days had a mean concentration > 50 $\mu g\ m^{-3}$. The risk for late neonatal mortality was 1.74 (95%; CI: 1.18-2.58, $p = 0.006$) when the concentration was 50 $\mu g\ m^{-3}$. On the days that the concentration exceeds 50 $\mu g\ m^{-3}$ the odds for late neonatal (8 to 28 days of life) mortality was 1.74 times higher than on days below this value. The shape of the association between PM and mortality does not show a threshold so it is suggested that even at lower concentrations the risk exists.	The study did not find significant associations between PM and mortality due to cardiorespiratory or SIDS causes, but significant associations were found in deaths due to perinatal circumstances. For late neonatal deaths the associations were significant with mortality due to congenital and chromosomal abnormalities.

Study	Study Location and Analyzed period	Methodology	Results	Interpretation
Son J, et. al. (2011)	Seoul Korea (2004-2007)	359,459 births with 225 deaths	Gestational PM concentrations were higher for infants who died compared to all normal-weight infants. The PM levels were similar across years with an annual average of 97.4 $\mu g\ m^{-3}$. They found associations between gestational exposure to all PM sizes and respiratory infant mortality; however, $PM_{2.5}$ alone specifically had statistical significance. Once exposed to TSP (total suspended particles), PM_{10} and $PM_{2.5}$ together were evaluated, and the risk for infant mortality was 3.78 (95%; CI: 1.50-25.66) and 3.15 (95%; CI: 1.26-7.85) respectively.	Air pollutants and particulate matter altogether have health consequences in infants as well as adults as shown by the TSP results alone. It is remarkable though that $PM_{2.5}$ alone also had statistically significant results if not for respiratory causes of death still it was a factor for other causes of infantile death.
Woodruff T, et al. (2008)	United States counties with >250,000 residents. (1999-2002).	3,583,495 births including 6,639 post-neonatal deaths in 96 counties.	Around 50% of infants died between 28 days and 3 months, 30% between 3 and 6 months and the remaining died between 6 months and 1 year of age. There were 576 deaths due to respiratory causes, 1379 due to SIDS, 755 due to ill-defined causes and 3, 622 due to other causes. There was a significant association between PM_{10} and $_{2.5}$ and respiratory death 16% (OR = 1.16; 95% CI: 1.06-1.27). The OR for increased quartiles of exposure was also significant since infants with high quartiles of exposure to $PM_{2.5}$ had an ele-vated R of respiratory mortality 1.39 (95%; CI: 1.04-1.61). Other causes of death did not have statistically significant association with $PM_{2.5}$.	Infantile death related to particulate matter seems to be related to the amount of exposure and the maturity of the infant. During the first year of life the biggest percentage of death was before 3 months (50%) which may suggest a higher risk to the pollutants due to a highly susceptible immune system.

The robust evidence about particulate matter and infant mortality found in different academic articles and done in different areas of the world strengthens the argument to update the WHO recommendation related to the threshold concentration of $PM_{2.5}$ currently allowed. In addition, there is evidence about this association in developed countries as well as developing countries. Some of the limitations of this paper is the lack of empirical data and the lack of control about the tools and data analysis done by each of the studies included in the review.

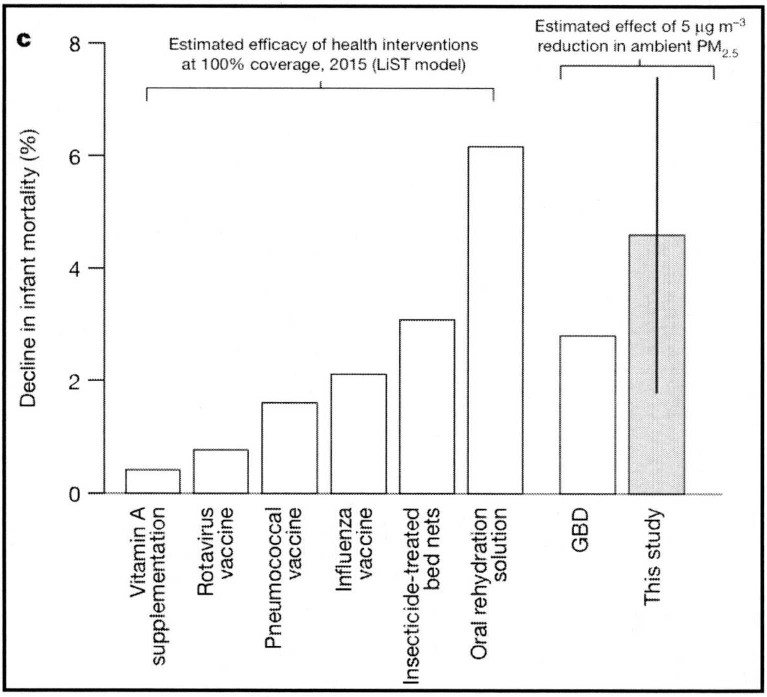

Figure 3. Comparison of estimated reductions in infant mortality if 100% coverage is achieved (11).

Conclusion

This literature review has shown that there is a strong correlation between the concentration of $PM_{2.5}$ in the environment and infant mortality. Two global studies were discussed in detail, and both show supporting findings. Other studies done in other areas of the world have also shown supportive evidence about the health risk air pollutants (particulate matter $_{2.5}$ being the focus) have on infantile health. Scheers et al. (12) argued that even in affluent areas of the world such as Western Europe, on days in which PM air pollution levels are high there is a significant correlation between concentration of PM and infant mortality (12).

Even in developed countries, which may have a marginal protective factor due to their usually lower concentration of $PM_{2.5}$, it is shown that due to seasonality and other ambient factors there is also a significant association between PM and infant death. In the study conducted by Heft-Neal et al. (11) the results show a similar correlation between infant mortality and $PM_{2.5}$ concentration in West Africa and the rest of Africa. According to the author, there is no evidence that wealth is a protective factor since the association between PM and mortality risk are similar across wealthy tertiles (11).

$PM_{2.5}$ generated by human activity significantly contributes to air pollution and negatively impacts human health. As this review shows, the association between infantile mortality and $PM_{2.5}$ is indisputable. In fact, according to Goyal, Karra and Canning (9) reducing carbonaceous $PM_{2.5}$ could contribute to reducing neonatal mortality to below 12 per 1000 children by 2030 (9). This evidence is pivotal and has relevant public health implications considering infant mortality across the globe could be reduced by promoting strategies to lower the levels of $PM_{2.5}$ in the air.

Moreover, the current World Health Organization guidelines limit the overall air concentration of $PM_{2.5}$ to 10 $\mu g\ m^{-3}$. However, there is evidence that naturally generated (dust and sea-salt) $PM_{2.5}$ and anthropogenic $PM_{2.5}$ have different effects on infant health and have shown to have the most destructive impact. It is therefore recommended that the WHO institute has different concentration thresholds for naturally produced PM and anthropogenic PM and establish new guidelines to lower the limit for anthropogenic $PM_{2.5}$ from the currently recommended 10 $\mu g\ m^{-3}$.

References

[1] World Health Organization. Ambient (outdoor) air pollution. Geneva: World Health Organization, 2018. URL: https://www.who.int/news-room/fact-sheets/detail/ambient-(outdoor)-air-quality-and-health.

[2] Greenstone M, Fan CQ. Introducing the air. URL: https://aqli.epic.uchicago.edu/wp-content/uploads/2018/11/AQLI-Intro-Report.pdf.

[3] Woodruff TJ, Darrow LA, Parker JD. Air pollution and post neonatal infant mortality in the United States, 1999–2002. Environ Health Perspect 2008;116(1):110–5.

[4] Centers for Disease Control and Prevention (CDC). Infant mortality. Atlanta, GA: CDC, 2020. URL: https://www.cdc.gov/reproductivehealth/maternalinfanthealth/infantmortality.html.

[5] Chen X, Shao S, Tian Z, Xie Z, Yin P. Impacts of air pollution and its Spatial spillover effect on public health based on China's big data sample. J Clean Product 2017;142:915–25.

[6] Malley CS, Kuylenstierna JC, Vallack HW, Henze DK, Blencowe H, Ashmore MR. Preterm birth associated with maternal fine particulate matter exposure: A global, regional, and national assessment. Environ Int 2017;101:173–82.

[7] Yorifuji T, Kashima S, Doi H. Acute exposure to fine and coarse particulate matter and infant mortality in Tokyo, Japan (2002–2013). Sci Total Environ 2016;551-552:66–72.

[8] Owili P, Lien WH, Muga M, Lin TH. The associations between types of ambient $pm_{2.5}$ and under-five and maternal mortality in Africa. Int J Environ Res Public Health 2017;14(4):359.

[9] Goyal N, Karra M, Canning D. Early-life exposure to ambient fine particulate air pollution and Infant mortality: Pooled evidence from 43 low- and middle-income countries. Int J Epidemiol 2019;48(4):1125–41.

[10] Son JY, Bell ML, Lee JT. Survival analysis of long-term exposure to different sizes of airborne particulate matter and risk of infant mortality using a birth cohort in Seoul, Korea. Environ Health Perspect 2011;119(5):725–30.

[11] Heft-Neal S, Burney J, Bendavid E, Burke M. Robust relationship between air quality and infant mortality in Africa. Nature 2018;559(7713):254–8.

[12] Scheers H, Mwalili SM, Faes C, Fierens F, Nemery B, Nawrot TS. Does air pollution trigger infant mortality in Western Europe? A case-crossover study. Environ Health Perspect 2011;119(7):1017–22.

Chapter 3

Pediatric prediabetes: Implications for adulthood

Thomas Pustorino[1], MD, MPH
Brigette Obokhae[1], MS
Jesmin Ram[1], BS
Jonathan Divito[1], BS
Gabriel Okenwa[1], BSc
Tolulope Oladimeji[2], MD, MPH
and Emmanuel O Keku[1], MD, MA, MSPH
[1]Department of Public Health and Preventive Medicine, St George's University, School of Medicine, St George, Grenada, West Indies
[2]Department of Pathophysiology, St George's University, School of Medicine, St George, Grenada, West Indies

Abstract

It is estimated that more than one-third of Americans have prediabetes and up to 18% of adolescents have diabetes or prediabetes. With the ever-rising obesity crisis worldwide, the prevalence of these conditions is rising in both children and adults, making it a significant public health concern. It is known that these high rates of diabetes place individuals at risk for several comorbid conditions such as renal failure and heart disease. However, the lasting effects of prediabetes in adolescents has been poorly described. Therefore, through a comprehensive literature review, it is the goal of this article to define what risk, if any, developing prediabetes as a child will have on their overall health as an adult. It is also a goal to see if these risks are similar to those who are diagnosed with diabetes as a child.

In: Public Health
Editors: Emmanuel O Keku and Joav Merrick
ISBN: 979-8-89113-083-8

Keywords: children, comorbidities, diabetes, pediatric, prediabetes, risk factors

Introduction

The increased prevalence of obesity within the pediatric population coincides with an increase in prediabetes, insulin resistance and diabetes (1). Diabetes is a group of metabolic diseases that are classified by hyperglycemia due to decreased insulin secretion, improper insulin action, or a combination of the two (20. However, before a patient is diagnosed with diabetes, they tend to develop an intermediate disease called prediabetes. Prediabetes is a serious condition defined as an asymptomatic prodromal period before developing diabetes, where an individual's plasma glucose levels are above the normally accepted range, but do not reach the threshold to be diagnosed with diabetes (3). It is estimated that "approximately 84 million Americans —more than 1 out of 3—have prediabetes" (4). This fact poses a large public health concern since 90% of individuals affected with prediabetes are unaware of their condition, placing them at risk of developing type 2 diabetes mellitus (T2DM), heart disease and stroke (4). Despite there being a wealth of knowledge regarding diabetes and prediabetes in adults, there is little evidence that exists regarding the pediatric population. Our current standards and knowledge on the topic of prediabetes in children is primarily information that is extrapolated from the adult population (1). This is specifically a pediatric public health concern considering that the prevalence of prediabetes is approximately 18% among adolescents and presentation of this condition at such a young age could expose this population to a high risk of long-term complications (5, 6). The TODAY Study, a randomized control study that examined children between the ages of 10-17 years, showed that children had a faster progression of T2DM and beta-cell failure as well as poorer response to treatment when comparing children to adults (7).

Therefore, the primary aim of this article is to identify the health risks of children who develop prediabetes and the distinct adverse effects, other than the known risks associated with adult diabetes, that individuals may be exposed to as a result of having prediabetes as a child. It is also the belief that there is a knowledge gap and lack of dedicated research in the field of prediabetes in children and that our known information is extrapolated from adults with diabetes.

Table 1. Selected articles, what databases were used in selecting them, and the general topic of the articles and how they relate to the research topic

Article	Database	Topic overview
Pathophysiology of prediabetes. Current Diabetes Reports	Google Scholar	Overview of prediabetes
Diagnosis and classification of diabetes mellitus	Google Scholar	Comparing effects of prediabetes to diabetes
Prevalence of prediabetes among adolescents and young adults in the United States	Google Scholar	Prevalence
Marked differences in prediabetes and diabetes associated comorbidities...	PubMed	Lifelong effects of prediabetes
Prediabetes—Your chance to prevent type 2 diabetes	Google Scholar	Overview of prediabetes
Obesity, physical activity and prediabetes in adult children of people with diabetes	NCBI	Lifelong effects of prediabetes
Prediabetes and cardiovascular parameters in obese children and adolescents	NCBI	Lifelong effects of prediabetes
Researching Effective Strategies to Improve Insulin Sensitivity in Children and Teenagers	PubMed	Treatment of prediabetes
Persistence of pre-diabetes in overweight and obese Hispanic children	Medscape	Lifelong effects of prediabetes
Addressing prediabetes in childhood obesity treatment programs	PubMed	Treatment of prediabetes
Metformin use in children and adolescents with prediabetes	NCBI	Treatment of prediabetes
Prevalence of prediabetes and type 2 diabetes in children with obesity	Medscape	Epidemiology of prediabetes
Prediabetes in children: Natural history, diagnosis, and preventive strategies	Google Scholar	Diagnosis/treatment of prediabetes
Effect of pre-diabetes on future risk of stroke	Google Scholar	Lifelong effects of prediabetes
Youth-onset type 2 diabetes mellitus: Lessons learned from the TODAY study	PubMed	Comparing effects of prediabetes to diabetes
Utility of hemoglobin a1c for diagnosing prediabetes and diabetes in obese children and adolescents	NCBI	Diagnosing prediabetes
Effect of regression from prediabetes to normal glucose regulation on long-term reduction in diabetes risk	Google Scholar	Lifelong effects of prediabetes
Prediabetes in children: What does it mean?	Medscape	Overview of prediabetes
Article	Database	Topic overview
Lower bone mass in prepubertal overweight children with prediabetes	NCBI	Lifelong effects of prediabetes
Prediabetes: The effects on arterial thickness and stiffness in obese youth	Google Scholar	Lifelong effects of prediabetes
Prediabetes in children and adolescents in the United States: Prevalence estimates and comorbidities	PubMed	Epidemiology of prediabetes
Identifying prediabetes and type 2 diabetes in asymptomatic youth	NCBI	Diagnosing prediabetes
Strategy for early identification of prediabetes in lean populations	NCBI	Diagnosing prediabetes
Prediabetes in obese youth: A syndrome of impaired glucose tolerance, severe insulin resistance, and altered myocellular and abdominal fat partitioning	PubMed	Overview/effects of prediabetes

Methods

To conduct a narrative review regarding the impact of childhood prediabetes on adult health, specific search criteria, databases, and inclusion and exclusion criteria were used to select supporting articles. Initial inclusion criteria consisted of children from all races and backgrounds between the ages of 10-18 years, who were diagnosed with prediabetes. These criteria served as the basis to establish the target sample. Exclusion criteria consisted of non-US citizens and the presence of comorbid conditions. Once a desired sample was established, specific keywords were selected to narrow the search for supporting articles. The following keywords were used to identify supporting articles: prediabetes, pediatric, children, comorbidities, diabetes, and risk factors. The following databases were used to search the selected keywords and obtain supporting articles: NCBI/PubMed, Google Scholar and Medscape. Only articles published in English were considered. The search was also limited to articles that had been published within the last 20 years; articles published beyond 20 years ago were not included.

Once the supporting articles were selected based upon the stated criteria, data was collected based on the age the children were initially diagnosed with prediabetes, whether they ever developed diabetes, and any conditions or adverse health effects they developed in their adult life. The data collected from the selected supporting articles was summarized and analyzed to draw a conclusion on the effects of prediabetes within the pediatric population on one's adult health.

Database search result

Applying the selected search criteria to the selected databases, 24 articles met the desired selection criteria and were included in the review. The selected articles discuss the topic of prediabetes in children in one way or another. Table 1 displays all the selected articles, what databases were used in selecting them, and the general topic of the articles and how they relate to the research topic.

Of the selected articles, 11 out of the 24 focused on the sole effect of having prediabetes as a child on one's adult life. These study designs consisted of a population cohort study, a cross-sectional study, retrospective and prospective cohort studies, meta-analysis, an observational study, population analysis and a randomized control trial. The majority of the articles focused on the most common side effects of diabetes, such as cardiovascular risk and stroke risk, while three articles focused on researching the unique side effects of childhood prediabetes on the developing body.

A cross sectional study conducted by the CDC concluded that the prevalence of prediabetes within the US was 18.0% among adolescents (95% CI, 16.0%-20.1%) and among young adults was 24.0% (95% CI, 22.0%-26.1%) (4). Andes et al. (5) equated these findings with a prevalence of a prediabetes diagnosis in 1 out of 5 adolescents and 1 out of 4 young. Male individuals and people with obesity were found to have a higher rate of prediabetes diagnoses.

Cardiovascular risk

Persistent prediabetes was shown to create an unfavorable cardiometabolic risk profile, putting children at an increased risk of type 2 diabetes as well as cardiovascular diseases (8, 9). This was shown to be a result of a declining metabolic profile that tended to result in a higher BMI, an increased systolic blood pressure, and elevated fasting insulin levels (9). As a result of this declining metabolic profile, individuals tended to have an increased incidence of dyslipidemia, hypertension and obesity in their adult lives further increasing their cardiovascular risk factors (10). In the study conducted by Andes et al. (5) it was found that adolescents and young adults with prediabetes had significantly higher non-HDL levels, higher systolic blood pressure, increased central adiposity, and lower insulin sensitivity ($P < .05$ for all) when compared to individuals without a diagnosis of prediabetes. A multivariate regression analysis was conducted during this study which found that prediabetes was a significant element of internal carotid intima media thickness and brachial distensibility ($P < .05$) Shah et al. (9) also found that after excluding youth diagnosed by HbA1C, the prediabetes group was significant, if not borderline, for internal carotid intima media thickness ($.1 > P \geq .05$).

Eklioğlu et al. (11) conducted a study looking at the direct effects that prediabetes has on the heart. Their results showed that left ventricular tissue doppler measurements were significantly higher in their prediabetes group. They also found that "left ventricular mass index (LVMi) was found to be positively correlated with triglyceride level, diastolic blood pressure, waist circumference, body weight standard deviation score and to negatively correlate with high-density lipoprotein cholesterol ($p = 0.043$, $r = 0.15$; $p = 0.039$, $r = 0.15$; $p = 0.025$, $r = 0.17$; $p = 0.009$, $r = 0.19$; $p = 0.038$, $r = -0.15$, respectively)." These findings are of great value since these negative metabolic states (e.g., high triglyceride level and low HDL) are the expected outcomes of having prediabetes over an extended period of time and would therefore correlate with an increase in left ventricular mass index. During this study a linear regression analysis was conducted that evaluated the cardiovascular risk factors of having prediabetes as a child. It was found that one's fasting glucose level was the best predictor of deterioration of cardiac function in prediabetic obese children and adolescents throughout the progression of their condition (11). These effects were even more prominent when compared to children without a diagnosis of prediabetes.

Stroke risk

In five out of the 15 prospective cohort studies that analyzed prediabetes conducted by Lee et al. (12), the random effects summary estimate showed an increased stroke risk after adjusting for established cardiovascular risk factors (1.21, 1.02 to 1.44; $P = 0.03$). Additionally, eight studies found that the random effects summary estimate for individuals with impaired glucose tolerance and impaired fasting glucose showed an increased risk of stroke after adjusting for established cardiovascular risk factors (1.26, 1.10 to 1.43; $P < 0.001$) (12).

Effect on bone growth

Pollock et al. (13) conducted a study looking at the effect that prediabetes has on bone health and development as a child. They found that the prediabetic individuals had a significantly lower total-body bone Mineral concentration (BMC) (1140.5 ± 15.7 versus 1182.5 ± 9.9 g, $p = .03$) as well as total-body bone area (1385.4 ± 9.4 versus 1410.8 ± 5.9 cm^2, $p = .03$) (13). Their findings suggested that abnormal glucose regulation as a result of a diagnosis of prediabetes may have a negative effect on one's developing bones prior to puberty and full growth.

General risks

Perreault et al. (14) aimed to calculate the diabetes risk in their Diabetes Prevention Program Outcomes Study (DPPOS). They found a 56% lower risk in developing diabetes in individuals who had returned to normal glucose regulation, if only transiently, versus those who consistently had prediabetes (hazard ratio [HR] 0·44, 95% CI 0·37–0·55, $p < 0{\cdot}0001$). They were also able to show that most of the variables that increase one's diabetic risk were inversely associated with the chance of a participant achieving a normal glucose range in the DPPOS. This was most evident with an increase in β-cell function (OR 1·28; 95% CI 1·18–1·39, $p < 0{\cdot}0001$) and insulin sensitivity (OR 1·16, 95% CI 1·08–1·25, $p < 0{\cdot}0001$) in individuals who were able to return to a normal glucose range (odds ratio [OR] 3·18, 95% CI 2·71–3·72, $p < 0{\cdot}0001$) (14). The study also concluded that the participants that did not return to a normal glycemic range, but were assigned to an intensive lifestyle modification, had a higher risk for developing diabetes in the future (HR 1·31, 95% CI 1·03–1·68, $p = 0{\cdot}0304$) and a lower chance of being able to successfully regulate there glucose levels (OR 0·59, 95% CI 0·42–0·82, $p = 0{\cdot}0014$) (14). This was in comparison to a placebo group within the study. Finally, the DPPOS concluded that prediabetes is a high-risk state for eventually developing diabetes. This was especially true in patients who persistently remained prediabetic despite intensive lifestyle modification. This in turn indicates that reversion to a normal and healthy glucose level, if only transiently, is associated with a significantly reduced risk of future diabetes and associated risk factors (14).

Diagnosis

The gold standard to diagnose diabetes as well as prediabetes is through the use of HbA1C and fasting glucose levels. Several selected studies evaluated how sensitive and specific these tests were in detecting prediabetes in children. Nowicka et al. (15) found that the standard use of an HbA1C of 6.5% would underestimate the prevalence of prediabetes and therefore should not be the sole measure used in order to diagnose the condition. Vajravelu et al. (16) found that HbA1C performs differently in children compared to adults. The test has a lower sensitivity for prediabetes (as low as 0–5% in children vs 23–27% in adults), a lower efficacy, and an even higher monetary cost.

Despite the high prevalence of prediabetes, a small number of patients are aware of their condition and are never officially diagnosed with prediabetes. Umapathi et al. (10) stated that "this reflects the lack of awareness among pediatricians about this underrecognized condition and its wide breadth of risk factors." Therefore, they proposed better screening and close follow up for this at-risk population to prevent its progression to diabetes as well as developing harmful risk factors. This is in lieu of the wide breadth of knowledge that is known about prediabetes and diabetes in the adult population. Umapathi et al. (10) also stated, "that there is paucity of data on this association in the pediatric population with regards to prediabetes."

Treatment

The standard of treatment for children with prediabetes is lifestyle modifications. Prediabetes is a complex health condition and modifications are best guided by a multidisciplinary team to address diet, exercise, psychological health, and other behavioral aspects in a culturally effective environment (1). Today there are no means of pharmacological treatments recommended. Khokhar et al. (17) conducted a study to determine if pharmacologically treating children with prediabetes would help improve their condition as well as help them lower their BMI. Through pediatric clinical trials, they found that the addition of metformin to lifestyle modifications further decreased BMI and improved glycemic control. Despite these beneficial results, they stated that most of the trials were of short duration with small sample sizes (17). As a result, it is recommended that more research be conducted to study the desired effects of metformin use in children.

Discussion

Analysis of the selected articles showed an emerging connection between prediabetes in children and adverse health effects in their adult lives. This connection became especially clear upon comparing children, who were diagnosed with prediabetes and a control group who did not have a diagnosis of prediabetes. Several articles also highlighted the adverse effects for children who remained prediabetic and never returned to a normal glycemic range.

The correlation between diabetes in both children and adults and adverse cardiovascular effects later in life is well known. However, Shah et al. (9) found a causal link between prediabetes in children and arterial thickness and stiffness. They concluded that adolescents with prediabetes also displayed cardiovascular changes consistent with early arterial disease. Furthermore, Lee et al. (12) concluded that there is an association between the diagnosis of prediabetes as a child and increased stroke risk.

Pollock et al. (13) compared bone mass in children with and without prediabetes and concluded that prediabetic children are at risk for poor skeletal development as well as central adiposity. They found that the "total-body bone mineral content was 4% lower in overweight children with prediabetes than in those without prediabetes after controlling for sex, race, height, and weight ($p = .03$) as well as an inverse relation with visceral adipose tissue ($\beta = -0.13$, $p = .03$) and subcutaneous abdominal adipose tissue ($\beta = -0.34$, $p = .02$) with bone mineral content after controlling for sex, race, and height" (13). This article emphasized a link between prediabetes in children and adverse health effects that are not traditionally seen in adults with diabetes or prediabetes.

Despite the conclusions drawn from these articles, there are several limitations. Firstly, many of these articles are over 10 years old and have a small sample size. This diminishes the power of the conclusions found within these studies and makes it difficult to apply them to the general population. Secondly, it was challenging to gain a comprehensive understanding of the adverse effects of childhood prediabetes on adult health due to the limited number of articles found.

There is also a knowledge gap in the current method for diagnosing prediabetes in children. It was found that the sole use of HbA1C does not accurately or reliably diagnose children with prediabetes, which could result in a missed or delayed diagnosis (15). Findings indicate that the inaccuracy of HbA1c as a diagnostic tool for prediabetic adolescents may serve as a barrier in preventing the development of diabetes in adulthood. HbA1c can be affected by a number of non-glycemic factors such as red blood cell turnover, hemoglobinopathies, medications, race, and age. In addition to its low sensitivity in children, HbA1c was found to function differently across diverse populations. For example, in Chinese populations HbA1c was a better indicator of prediabetes compared to the impaired fasting glucose (IFG) test (77% for HbA1c vs 27.7% for IFG), whereas in US populations, it is the opposite (24.8% for HbA1c vs 80.1% for fasting plasma glucose - FPG) (16). However, one article suggested that among young and lean populations, having a high blood glucose level poses a future risk of prediabetes/diabetes

(18). Further investigation on the role of HbA1c's diagnostic capabilities of prediabetes in children is required as well as a potential alternative diagnostic tool that could more reliably diagnose the condition.

These articles also highlighted additional barriers that should be considered when diagnosing and treating prediabetic adolescents. Socioeconomic status and the family dynamic were shown to be a social determinant that could have a negative effect on the development of diabetes. Compeán-Ortiz et al. (19) found that 64% of children with parents that had been diagnosed with diabetes had a BMI in the overweight/obesity range, and with consideration to waist circumference, 73.6% had abdominal obesity and 68% had an increased or substantially increased risk for cardiovascular diseases (17).

Compeán-Ortiz et al. (13) stated that "obesity and [being] overweight are prediabetes condition[s], whose etiology have a double association with the family organization: the genetic inheritance imposes a dominant element on the transmission of DM2, and eating habits and physical activities that are modulated within the family group." These findings suggest that diabetes is a familial concern. Hence, health professionals should consider preventative interventions that can be practiced by the entire family unit, such as lifestyle modifications that include healthier eating habits and increased physical activity, when determining the treatment plans for people diagnosed with diabetes.

The incidence and prevalence of prediabetes has been exacerbated by sedentary lifestyles, high caloric diets, obesity and hepatic-related diseases (20). While there is a considerable difference in the incidence and prevalence of pediatric T2DM amongst specific age and ethnic/racial groups, Haemer et al. (1) emphasized the importance of providing all pre-diabetic youth access to a multidisciplinary team, including a behavioral health professional, endocrinologist, exercise specialist and nutritionist. Clinical studies have found that youth with T2DM have high rates of psychiatric diagnoses, which requires persistent surveillance of mental and behavioral health. Studies have also linked depressive symptomatology to the development of insulin resistance in youth. Behavioral health professionals are an important asset to providing culturally sensitive pediatric healthcare to address adherence barriers such as comorbid psychopathologies, medical compliance, and familial dynamics. Given the high incidence of T2DM and familial dynamics, focusing behavioral treatment on the entire family unit of youth with prediabetes or T2DM may be necessary (1).

While there is no single approved diet for diabetes prevention in youth, clinical studies have shown that a low glycemic diet can improve insulin secretion, body weight and body composition (1, 21). However, youth from racial and ethnic minority groups, low socioeconomic status, and single-parent families are more likely to experience food insecurity (i.e., access to stores that sell the foods recommended in lifestyle modification plans and the ability to afford those food items), in addition to, lack of access to appropriate multidisciplinary healthcare, and medical noncompliance with their chronic diseases (1).

We believe that addressing these barriers would reduce the prevalence of prediabetes in children thus reducing the risk of developing diabetes in adulthood. The amount of evidence and research on preventing the progression of prediabetes and successfully mitigating its negative outcomes is very limited. There is a need for further independent research with larger sample sizes to assess the impact of childhood prediabetes on adult health.

Conclusion

With the ever-growing obesity crisis, children are developing prediabetes and diabetes at increasing rates. The studies included in this review have shown that being diagnosed with prediabetes as a child can adversely affect adult health. These adverse effects include the expected comorbidities of diabetes, such as cardiovascular risks and increased stroke risk, as well as the unique consequences of childhood prediabetes such as decreased bone mineral density, increased arterial thickening and stiffening, and an increased risk of developing diabetes and a poor metabolic profile. The selected articles have shown that prediabetes itself is a serious condition that requires adequate diagnosis and treatment to improve patient health. It is recommended that future research be conducted on all aspects of prediabetes in children to acquire a better understanding of the potential adverse health effects, diagnostic measures.

References

[1] Haemer MA, Grow HM, Fernandez C, Lukasiewicz GJ, Rhodes ET, Shaffer LA, Estrada E. Addressing prediabetes in childhood obesity treatment programs: Support from research and current practice. Child Obes 2014;10(4):292–303.

[2] ADA. Diagnosis and classification of diabetes mellitus. Diab Care 2006;29(Suppl 1):S43-48.

[3] Pinhas-Hamiel O, Zeitler P. Prediabetes in children: What does it mean? Medscape 2013 Jan 02.

[4] Centers for Disease Control and Prevention. Prediabetes: Your chance to prevent type 2 diabetes. Atlanta, GA: National Center for Chronic Disease Prevention and Health Promotion, Division of Diabetes Translation, 2021.

[5] Andes LJ, Cheng YJ, Rolka DB,Gregg EW,Imperatore G. Prevalence of prediabetes among adolescents and young adults in the United States, 2005-2016. JAMA Pediatr 2020;174(2):e194498.

[6] Weiss R, Dufour S, Taksali SE, Tamborlane WV, Petersen KF, Bonadonna RC, et al. Prediabetes in obese youth: A syndrome of impaired glucose tolerance, severe insulin resistance, and altered myocellular and abdominal fat partitioning. Lancet 2003;362(9388):951–7.

[7] Narasimhan S, Weinstock RS. Youth-onset type 2 diabetes mellitus: Lessons learned from the TODAY study. Mayo Clinic Proceedings 2014;89(6):806–16.

[8] Abdul-Ghani MA, DeFranzo RA. Pathophysiology of prediabetes. Curr Diab Rep 2009;9(3):193–9.

[9] Shah AS, Gao Z, Urbina EM, Kimball TR, Dolan LM. Prediabetes: The effects on arterial thickness and stiffness in obese youth. J Clin Endocrinol Metabol 2014;99(3):1037–43.

[10] Umapathi KK, Thavamani A, Al-Kindi S. Prediabetes in children and adolescents in the United States: Prevalence estimates and comorbidities - A population analysis. J Pediatr Endocrinol Metabol 2019;32(2):187–9.

[11] Eklioğlu BS, Atabek ME, Akyürek N, Alp H. Prediabetes and cardiovascular parameters in obese children and adolescents. J Clin Res Pediatr Endocrinol 2016;8(1):80–5.

[12] Lee M, Saver JL, Hong KS, Song S, Chang KH, Ovbiagele B. Effect of pre-diabetes on future risk of stroke: Meta-analysis. BMJ 2012;344:e3564.

[13] Pollock NK, Bernard PJ, Wenger K, Misra S, Gower BA, Allison JD et al. Lower bone mass in prepubertal overweight children with prediabetes. J Bone Mineral Res 2010;25(12):2760–9.

[14] Perreault L, Pan Q, Mather KJ, Watson KE, Hamman RF, Kahn SE. Effect of regression from prediabetes to normal glucose regulation on long-term reduction in diabetes risk: Results from the Diabetes Prevention Program Outcomes Study. Lancet 2012;379(9833):2243–51.

[15] Nowicka P, Santoro N, Liu H, Lartaud D, Shaw MM, Goldberg R et al. Utility of hemoglobin A1c for diagnosing prediabetes and diabetes in obese children and adolescents. Diab Care 2011;34(6):1306–11.

[16] Vajravelu ME, Lee JM. Identifying prediabetes and type 2 diabetes in asymptomatic youth: Should HbA1c be used as a diagnostic approach? Curr Diab Rep 2018;18(7):43.

[17] Khokhar A, Umpaichitra V, Chin VL, Perez-Colon S. Metformin use in children and adolescents with prediabetes. Pediatr Clin North Am 2017;64(6):1341–53.

[18] Wang G, Radovick S, Xu X, Xing H, Tang G, Bartell TR, et al. Strategy for early identification of prediabetes in lean populations: New insight from a prospective Chinese twin cohort of children and young adults. Diab Res Clin Pract 2018;146:101–10.

[19] Compeán-Ortiz LG, Trujillo-Olivera LE, Valles-Medina AM, Reséndiz-González E, García-Solano B, Pérez BDA. Obesity, physical activity, and prediabetes in adult children of people with diabetes. Rev Latino-Americana Enfermagem 2018;25:e2981.

[20] Koutny F, Weghuber D, Bollow E, Greber-Platzer S, Hartmann K, Körner A et al. Prevalence of prediabetes and type 2 diabetes in children with obesity and increased transaminases in European German-speaking countries. Analysis of the APV initiative. Pediatr Obes 2020;15(4):e12601.

[21] Garnett SP, Baur LA, Noakes M, Steinbeck K, Woodhead HJ, Burrell S et al. Researching Effective Strategies to Improve Insulin Sensitivity in Children and Teenagers—RESIST. A randomized control trial investigating the effects of two different diets on insulin sensitivity in young people with insulin resistance and/or pre-diabetes. BMC Public Health 2010;10(1):575.

Chapter 4

The benefits of cardiac rehabilitation for the prevention of second myocardial infarction and the effects of underutilization based on socioeconomic status

Ian Mathies[1], MPH
Giovanni Paolella Jr[1], MA
Camden Fuller[1], MSE
Stacia Verrett[1], MPH
Anthony La[1], BA
Vanessa Osei-Bonsu[1], BS
Tolulope Oladimeji[2], MD, MPH
and Emmanuel O Keku[1], MD, MA, MSPH
[1]Department of Public Health and Preventive Medicine, St George's University, School of Medicine, St George, Grenada, West Indies
[2]Department of Pathophysiology, St George's University, School of Medicine, St George, Grenada, West Indies

Abstract

The occurrence of a second myocardial infarction (MI) and the quality of life in cardiac rehabilitation (CR) patients was compared to those with a prior MI in the community setting. The accessibility of rehab facilities and the population who utilize them were also investigated the link between lower SES, CR and mortality post-MI. Methods: The study was conducted using search engines such as Google Scholar, PubMed,

In: Public Health
Editors: Emmanuel O Keku and Joav Merrick
ISBN: 979-8-89113-083-8

Science Direct, and Medline Plus. Each article was published within the last 5 to 10 years, except for hallmark papers for background information. 10 articles were analyzed, and 15 supporting articles were included in this study. Finally, 46 articles were reviewed, to the argument or provided evidence contrary to current beliefs.

The effects of CR have significant benefits for patients after an acute MI, ranging from reducing the risk of a second MI, to improving their quality of life. Despite all the proven benefits of CR, there is only a 35% participation for patients post-acute MI. Furthermore, people of low SES have greater risk factors for acute MI, a higher first-time incidence rate, less access to CR, and lower CR attendance rates. More effort must be placed into expanding the general accessibility of CR, better education for cardiac patients on the benefits, and access to easier and affordable alternatives to onsite CR.

Keywords: myocardial infarction, cardiac rehabilitation, socioeconomic status, cardiovascular disease, cardiovascular risk factors, prevention, preventative medicine, public health

Introduction

Cardiovascular disease is the leading cause of death in the United States and one of the top causes of death worldwide (1). According to the American Heart Association, about 17.8 million deaths in 2017 were attributed to cardiovascular disease; for myocardial infarction (MI) alone, there are 1.5 million new cases in the United States each year (2). There are a multitude of factors that can lead to cardiovascular disease, including diet, body mass index (BMI), physical activity, family history, socioeconomic status, quality of sleep, occupation, and chronic stress levels (3).

According to a study by Gerber et al. (4), MI recurrence happens in about 27.5% of MI patients and leads to an increased risk of mortality compared to an initial MI, with a hazard ratio of 1.49. A comparison of the outcomes of post-MI patients who had cardiac rehab and post-MI patients in the community will be made. We hypothesized that post-MI patients in the community will have higher occurrence of a second of MI, higher mortality rates, and lower quality of life compared to those in cardiac rehab. Furthermore, it was anticipated that individuals of lower socioeconomic status will have a higher rate of second incidence of MI and higher mortality rates. For those who are aware of the benefits of optimal exercise and diet, motivation may also play a significant role in the outcomes of post-MI patients who do not attend rehab compared to those in the rehab group.

Preventative measures: How rehabilitation is designed to prevent a second MI

Following an MI, a patient will need a certain amount of rest to recover from the initial damage before starting any physical activity. The length of the rest period, the frequency, duration, and type of activity will depend on the patient (5). Hence, patients undergo evaluation before commencing cardiac rehab and discovery of significant comorbidity might result in exclusion from cardiac rehab. For instance, the European Society of Cardiology, posited that a patient would be temporarily excluded from exercise consideration if unstable angina were present (6). Patient are risk stratified into low, moderate, and high risk based on variables from a twelve-lead resting EKG testing, resting echocardiography, classical exercise testing or Cardiopulmonary Stress Test (CPX), assessment of cardiovascular risk factors, and an exam of the pulmonary and osteoarticular systems.

During this structured rehabilitation, the most used parameter for training level is heart rate. To determine a patient's target heart rate, the Karvonen formula is used. The heart rate must be between 60 to 70% of the Karvonen formula which is calculated based on the individual's maximal and resting heart rate, both of which are calculated from the person's age. This helps to standardize treatment for patients based on age; however, cardiac arrythmias are major limitations to this (6).

When a person survives a myocardial infarction, it is typically recommended that they attend cardiac rehabilitation. The details mentioned above depict how these patients are closely monitored to ensure they are not straining themselves while also holding the patient accountable for their exercises. Due to the multifactorial nature of the rehab process, it is also universally understood by cardiologists that an individualized workout routine should be created to meet the specific needs of each patient. However, in a study conducted by Stromback et al. (7), they address how many patients felt that their rehab should have been more customized to their condition and prognosis, and they did not perceive their care was individualized. The patient's perception of treatment efficacy is a crucial factor that should be considered when trying to encourage MI patients to take advantage of the benefits offered by participating in cardiac rehab.

Methods

Literature database search involved the use of Google Scholar and the following databases: PubMed, Science Direct, Medline Plus, and Hinari. All studies included were published within the last 10 years unless the source was used to explain undisputed information on a subject and supply background information necessary to introduce new ideas and theories still being tested. Information was determined to be credible if it came from a scientific journal, publication, or trusted public health organization such as the World Health Organization or Center for Disease Control.

While searching for articles, lists of phrases were made that were used to find the selected articles. If a study was found to have significant value towards our objective, then it was added to a list using Mendeley, thoroughly critiqued and incorporated into the paper. Some of the key search phrases that were used included "effect of exercise on patients with history of myocardial infarction," "optimal exercise for patients with heart problems," "rehabilitation for MI patients," "preventative care for patients with history of MI," "prevalence of myocardial infarction in the United States," "slow gait speed and myocardial infarction rehabilitation," "heart rate zone in myocardial infarction rehabilitation," "heart rate zone in myocardial infarction rehabilitation in rehab centers," "second occurrence of myocardial infarction in cardiac rehabilitation patients," "how do you pay for cardiac rehab," and "prevalence of myocardial infarction in the US for patients who do not go to cardiac rehabilitation."

If the information seemed to be theory-based or in early development, then other articles were found that could either support or contradict this new information to improve its validity. 10 studies were analyzed, and 15 supporting articles were used, making a total of 25 sources that were included in this study. Finally, though 46 articles were analyzed, they were only included if they contained statistically significant data that contributed to the argument or provided evidence that contradicted current beliefs. During the analysis, results were described from each paper and how they contribute to the argument. It was then discussed whether there were any gaps in information that could be further studied and included.

Analysis

The benefits of cardiac rehabilitation after a myocardial infarction include decreased mortality rate, decreased recurrence rate of future MIs, and improved quality of life. In a study by Zhang et al. (8), they demonstrated this in a randomized control trial with 130 STEMI patients following percutaneous coronary intervention (PCI). The patients were divided into two groups of 65 people each, with the intervention group participating in rehabilitation while the control group did not. The tests conducted on the participants were cardiac function test, a 6-minute walk test, determination of capability of exercise, and cardiac risk factors, measured both before and after the rehab period. The intervention group showed fewer recurrences of angina and hospital readmission rates, as well as a greater improvement in ventricular ejection fraction.

Furthermore, a randomized control study by Lee et al. (9) used an exercise tolerance test and a quality-of-life assessment questionnaire on acute MI patients who recently underwent PCI. Of the 122 participants, 72 attended cardiac rehabilitation, while 50 did not. Testing and surveys were administered to all patients two weeks after their PCI, which was the participants' first visit to the Cardiac Health Rehabilitation Center. Both groups were then re-evaluated two months later, and it was found that the rehab group had statistically significant improvements in physical functioning, body pain, general health perceptions, social role functioning, and mental health, as well as improved quality-of-life and overall physical ability. Therefore, cardiac rehab plays a vital role in the reduction of stress levels for its participants, putting them at a decreased risk for a future MI.

Doimo et al. (10) using a multivariable regression model explored the long-term benefits of cardiac rehabilitation, they analyzed the 5-year incidence of cardiovascular mortality and hospitalization resulting from cardiovascular disease, comparing those who attended ambulatory cardiac rehab and those who did not. The study revealed that cardiovascular related mortality rate was 18% in the rehab group compared to 30% in the control group over a 5-year period. There were also only 15% cardiac-related hospitalizations from the rehab group compared to 27% in the control group (10).

Cardiac rehabilitation and accessibility to patients

According to the American Heart Association, most health insurance provides reimbursement for cardiac rehabilitation, for example, Medicare covers two one-hour sessions per day for up to 32 session (11). However, in 2018, the United States Census Bureau reported that 8.5% of Americans, (27.5 million people), did not have health insurance, an increase from 7.9% (25.6 million people) in 2017 (12). This shows a downward trend in the number of people that have financial coverage for cardiac rehabilitation. In an article published in 2001 by the Institute of Medicine, people are most likely to have insurance coverage if they are employed full-time or have a moderate level annual income (greater than 200% of the federal poverty level) (13). Furthermore, "two-thirds of all uninsured persons are members of lower-income families (earning less than 200% of the federal poverty level). One-third of all members of lower income families are uninsured" (13). Therefore, in the US, most people that are not insured for cardiac rehabilitation are of low SES, which makes up almost 10% of the population, and is growing every year.

Though most insurance covers rehab, is more expensive, multidisciplinary CR more effective? Though most insurance companies cover some form of cardiac rehabilitation following acute MI, it raises the question: are all rehab programs of equal quality? In a retrospective cohort study by Ogawa et al. (14), they demonstrate that compared to conventional exercise-based rehab, a multidisciplinary approach resulted in significantly lower unplanned readmission rate, with a hazard ratio of 0.520 using a multivariable regression analysis. Therefore, a more well-rounded rehab program that concentrates on exercise, as well as diet, positive lifestyle choices and mental health results in far fewer hospital readmissions. It is worth studying which health insurers do and do not cover this variety of rehabilitation.

Most common demographics of MI patients that attend cardiac rehabilitation

Despite the significant benefits of cardiac rehab, in 2017 the Center for Disease Control (CDC) reported that only 34% of people with heart failure used rehab services, and only 36% of heart attack survivors were enrolled in programs (15). Therefore, patients are underutilizing these facilities, even when the programs are accessible. The study conducted by the CDC also concluded that among the 9,490 MI patients that were studied, "older adults, men, non-Hispanic whites, persons with college or higher education, and those with two, three, or four (of five) CVD risk factors were more likely to receive cardiac rehab than were younger persons, women, non-Hispanic blacks, Hispanics, persons with less than a college education, and persons with fewer than two or with five CVD risk factors" (15). Not only were white, but non-Hispanics also utilizing rehab significantly more than Black, non-Hispanic people and Hispanic people (35.4% compared to 25.3%, respectively), as the level of patient education increased, so did their likelihood of participating in cardiac rehab. For the percentage of rehab participation based on level of education: less than high school diploma was 23.3%, high school diploma was 36.1%, some college was 33.0%, and college graduate was 46.4% participation.

This shows that the level of education has a significant influence on an individual's decision to attend cardiac rehab following an MI. This lack of participation may indicate that many patients are unaware of the benefits of rehab following an MI, and efforts should be made by practitioners to improve enrollment, as well as improve utilization of at home-based therapies. However, for homeless individuals, these at-home physical therapies are inaccessible and proper dieting is also unattainable; therefore, enrollment of such individuals to an onsite facility would be essential.

Cardiac rehabilitation and socioeconomic status: Accessibility and smoking

Not only are the attendance rates for cardiac rehabilitation much lower for MI patients of lower SES, but a study in Finland by Salomaa et al. (16) analyzed the FINMONICA MI Registrar of all MI events among men and women between the ages of 35 and 64 years. When comparing the initial incidence rates of MI, the rate ratios of lower-income and middle-income individuals were 1.67 and 1.84 respectively, when compared with high-income individuals (16). Therefore, not only are lower-SES patients less likely to attend cardiac rehab, they are also at a greater risk for an initial heart attack. The study goes on to say that the 28-day and 1-year mortality rate ratios of MI patients in lower- and middle-income individuals were 3.18 and 2.33 compared to high-income individuals, which is likely due in part to differences in cardiac rehabilitation participation rates between the three groups (16).

Exploring a study conducted by Borg et al. (17), a logistic regression analysis was used to analyze 31,297 patients who suffered an acute MI –

specifically with the variable of whether cardiac rehab was utilized. They showed that the strongest predictor for non-attendance was the inconvenient distance traveled from home to the nearest cardiac facility, where participants were 1.75 times less likely to make that travel compared to those who's distance was more convenient. Smoking, a high burden of comorbidities, and employment status were also predictors of non-attendance (17). When looking at these predictors, it is likely that we can correlate them to poor living conditions secondary to being of low socioeconomic status. It is not uncommon for low-SES areas to be out-of-reach from vital resources, such as good-quality hospitals, putting this group at a disadvantage for receiving rehab because it is either not convenient to attend or they simply do not have the means of transportation to get there. It is also worth noting that smoking is far more prevalent in low-SES individuals – smoking twice as many pack-years compared to high-SES individuals (18). Low SES individuals are also at a greater risk of suffering from a greater number of comorbidities and are forced to work longer hours, all of which were predictors of non-attendance in this study (19).

People of low-SES have a greater number of risk factors for acute MI prior to their first MI. But according to a study by Gaalema et al. (20), which observed the effect of SES on the propensity to change risk factors following infarct, lower-SES patients were 2 to 4 times less likely to change their lifestyle and modify risk factors following an MI. The authors studied smoking cessation, cardiac rehab, medication adherence, diet, and physical activity. They concluded that initiatives to increase participation in cardiac rehabilitation or other secondary prevention programs should be a priority, as they address multiple behaviors that increase the risk of a subsequent MI. It is possible that once habits are managed in these patients, the risk of a second MI will be reduced along with the risk of developing many other comorbidities that affect this low-SES population, such as diabetes mellites.

Effect of awareness on the use of cardiac rehabilitation post-MI

A study by Josephson and Mahenna (21) explained that even though many cardiologists appreciate the benefits of primary and secondary prevention of cardiovascular disease, they are ineffective in getting this message across to their patients. Many give vague instructions, such as only telling patients to exercise more, when they should be using the same level of detail used in writing a pharmaceutical prescription, stating details like the dose and frequency. A useful recommended framework for physicians to prescribe exercise to a patient uses the acronym FITT, which stands for Frequency, Intensity, Time, and Type of exercise. This framework should be used for post-MI patients since such a low percentage utilize cardiac rehab services, and it is becoming apparent that alternatives, such as at-home therapy, telemedicine, and yoga, should be emphasized. This may help create more equity in rehab care among post-MI patients of different income levels to account for the disparities that occur in individuals with low SES and those that lack higher-level education.

Limitations

There is limited research that specifically focuses on the effects of cardiac rehabilitation on the occurrence of a second myocardial infarction; therefore, we also looked at readmission and mortality rates as proxy measures for MI recurrence.

Conclusion

Cardiac rehabilitation has significant benefits for patients with acute myocardial infarction, such as reduction in the risk of a second myocardial infarction and improving quality-of-life. Despite all these benefits, 35% of patient participates in cardiac rehab following an acute myocardial infarction. Furthermore, people of low SES have greater risk factors for acute MI, a higher first-time incidence rate, and have less access to cardiac rehab treatment. When these patients do have access to treatment, they have lower attendance rates compared to those with higher SES. There needs to be more efforts in expanding the general accessibility of cardiac rehabilitation to this population, as well as a need for better education to all cardiac patients on the benefits of attending. Finally, emphasis should be placed on ways of accessing the benefits of cardiac rehab without attending onsite, making it easier and more affordable to attend.

Recommendations

The lack of participation in cardiac rehab is a significant public health problem. A study by Ades et al. (22) on increasing cardiac rehab participation from 20% to 70% describes a road map designed by the Million Hearts initiative to prevent 1 million cardiovascular events over five years. The researchers anticipate that achieving this goal would save 25,000 lives and prevent 180,000 hospitalizations in the US annually. They plan to utilize electronic medical record-based prompts and staffing liaisons to increase the number of referrals to cardiac rehab centers to those that would benefit. Though this does not focus strictly on the low-SES individuals, if initiatives like this are successful at increasing attendance rates and highlighting the benefits of these services, then people in the low-SES areas may be more aware of the benefits and be incentivized to go when they have the access.

Alternatives for rehabilitation that could be beneficial at the community level

At-home cardiac rehabilitation

For patients that live too far from a facility or lack adequate transportation, Kraal et al. discuss one way in which on-site services can be substituted by an at home-based therapy (16, 23). Through a randomized control trial of 90 low-to-moderate risk patients, differences between a home-based telemonitored cardiac rehab and onsite rehab were measured. The study concluded that there was no significant difference in the physical fitness or quality of life in the two groups following therapy, but the home-based cardiac rehab was more cost-effective and had a higher level of patient satisfaction. Therefore, telemedicine may be an alternative for patients in any demographic. This also allows patients to complete their therapy in situations mandating stay at home orders, such as those seen during the COVID-19 pandemic or extreme weather conditions.

Yoga-based therapy

Another viable variation to cardiac rehabilitation is a yoga-based cardiac rehabilitation. A study was performed in India by Chandrasekaran et al. motivated by the high prevalence of low-SES cardiac patients in the country, proposed the use of yoga as a more cost-effective and accessible form of therapy and are currently studying its effectiveness on post-MI patients (24).

Family support

Finally, it is worth mentioning that one's family and social support systems play a significant role in a patient's prognosis and recovery. Though the study did not provide enough in its findings to be validated, Vahedian-Azimi et al. (25) sought to compare the standard cardiac rehab therapy against a cardiac rehab with a Family Centered Empowerment Model. Further research should be done to examine the effects of family support on therapy outcomes, and if those without family have an increased incidence of MI reoccurrence, rehospitalization, and higher mortality rates.

Further studies on cardiac rehabilitation are vital because it is an accessible and effective tool that can protect against the leading cause of death throughout the world. Proper patient education about cardiac rehab as well as suggesting alternative forms of individualized rehab that better fit the patient's lifestyle will reduce the recurrence risk of acute myocardial infarction and other cardiac disorders, thereby creating equity in the treatment of patients with heart conditions.

References

[1] Sidney S, Sorel ME, Quesenberry CP, Jaffe MG, Solomon MD, Nguyen-Huynh MN, et al. Comparative trends in heart disease, stroke, and all-cause mortality in the United States and a large integrated healthcare delivery system. Am J Medicine 2018;131(7):829-36.

[2] Benjamin EJ, Muntner P, Alonso A, Bittencourt MS, Callaway CW, Carson AP, et al. Heart disease and stroke statistics—2019 update: A report from the American Heart Association. Circulation 2019;139(10):e56-28.

[3] Dodson JA, Geda M, Krumholz HM, Lorenze N, Murphy TE, Allore HG, et al. Design and rationale of the comprehensive evaluation of risk factors in older patients with AMI (SILVER-AMI) study. BMC Health Serv Res 2014;14(1):1-9.

[4] Gerber Y, Weston SA, Jiang R, Roger VL. The changing epidemiology of myocardial infarction in Olmsted County, Minnesota, 1995-2012. Am J Medicine 2015;128(2):144-51.

[5] Bahall M, Khan K. Quality of life of patients with first time AMI: A descriptive study. Health Qual Life Outcomes 2018;16(1):1-10.

[6] Carre F. Whether and how to establish an exercise plan in cardiac patients. E-Journal Cardiol Pract 2010;9:1.

[7] Strömbäck U, Wälivaara BM, Vikman I, Lundblad D, Engström Å. To be seen as a unique person after suffering a second myocardial infarction: Expressed needs of patients and descriptions of personnel. Intensive Crit Care Nurs 2020;57:102797

[8] Zhang Y, Cao H, Jiang P, Tang H. Cardiac rehabilitation in acute myocardial infarction patients after percutaneous coronary intervention: A community-based study. Medicine 2018;97(8):e9785.

[9] Lee BJ, Go JY, Kim AR, Chun SM, Park M, Yang DH, Park HS, Jung TD. Quality of life and physical ability changes after hospital-based cardiac rehabilitation in patients with myocardial infarction. Ann Rehab Med 2017;41(1):121.

[10] Doimo S, Fabris E, Piepoli M, Barbati G, Canterin F, Bernardi G, Maras P, Sinagra Impact of ambulatory cardiac rehabilitation on cardiovascular outcomes: a long-term follow-up study. Eur Heart J 2019;40(8):678-85. URL: https://doi.org/10.1093/eurheartj/ehy417.

[11] American Heart Association. Am I eligible for cardiac rehab? URL: https://www.heart.org/en/health-topics/cardiac-rehab/am-i-eligible-for-cardiac-rehab.

[12] Berchick ER, Barnett JC, Upton RD. Health insurance coverage in the United States: 2018. Suitland-Silver Hill, MD: United States Census Bureau, Report, 2019.

[13] Institute of Medicine (US) Committee on the Consequences of Uninsurance. Coverage matters: Insurance and health care. Washington, DC: National Academies Press, 2001.

[14] Ogawa M, Satomi S, Yoshida N, Tsuboi Y, Komaki K, Wakida K, et al. Effects of acute-phase multidisciplinary rehabilitation on unplanned readmission after cardiac surgery. J Thorac Cardiovasc Surg 2021;161(5):1853-60.

[15] Fang J, Ayala C, Luncheon C, Ritchey M, Loustalot F. Use of outpatient cardiac rehabilitation among heart attack survivors—20 states and the District of Columbia, 2013 and four states, 2015. MMWR 2017;66(33):869.

[16] Salomaa V, Niemelä M, Miettinen H, Ketonen M, Immonen-Räihä P, Koskinen S, Mähönen M, Lehto S, Vuorenmaa T, Palomäki P, Mustaniemi H. Relationship of socioeconomic status to the incidence and prehospital, 28-day, and 1-year mortality rates of acute coronary events in the FINMONICA myocardial infarction register study. Circulation 2000;101(160;1913-8.

[17] Borg S, Öberg B, Leosdottir M, Lindolm D, Nilsson L, Bäck M. Factors associated with non-attendance at exercise-based cardiac rehabilitation. BMC Sports Sci Med Rehabil 2019;11(1):1-0.

[18] Center for Disease Control. Cigarette smoking and tobacco use among people of low socioeconomic status. Atlanta, GA: Centers for Disease Control and Prevention, 2019. URL. https://www.cdc.gov/tobacco/disparities/low-ses/index.htm.

[19] Suwannaphant K, Laohasiriwong Puttana pon N, Saengsuwan J, Phajan T. Association between socioeconomic status and diabetes mellitus: The national socioeconomics survey, 2010-2012. J Clin Diagn Res 2017;11(7):LC18-22. doi: 10.7860/JCDR/2017/28221.10286.

[20] Gaalema DE, Elliott RJ, Morford ZH, Higgins ST, Ades PA. Effect of socioeconomic status on propensity to change risk behaviors following myocardial infarction: implications for healthy lifestyle medicine. Progr Cardiovasc Dis 2017;60(1):159-68.

[21] Josephson RA, Mehanna E. Exercise prescription: The devil is in the details. Am Coll Cardiol 2016 Feb 11.

[22] Ades PA, Keteyian SJ, Wright JS, Hamm LF, Lui K, Newlin K, Shepard DS, Thomas RJ. Increasing cardiac rehabilitation participation from 20% to 70%: A road map from the million hearts cardiac rehabilitation collaborative. Mayo Clin Proceed 2017;92(2):234-42.

[23] Kraal JJ, Van den Akker-Van Marle ME, Abu-Hanna A, Stut W, Peek N, Kemps HM. Clinical and cost-effectiveness of home-based cardiac rehabilitation compared to conventional, centre-based cardiac rehabilitation: Results of the FIT@ Home study. Eur J Prev Cardiol 2017;24(12):1260-73.

[24] Prabhakaran D, Chandrasekaran AM, Singh K, Mohan B, Chattopadhyay K, Chadha DS et al. Yoga-based cardiac rehabilitation after acute myocardial infarction: a randomized trial. J Am Coll Cardiol 2020;75(13):1551-61.

[25] Vahedian-Azimi A, Miller A, Hajiesmaieli M, Kangasniemi M, Alhani F, Jelvehmoghaddam H et al. Cardiac rehabilitation using the family-centered empowerment model versus home-based cardiac rehabilitation in patients with myocardial infarction: A randomized controlled trial. Open Heart 2016;3(1): e000349. doi:10.1136/openhrt-2015-000349.

Chapter 5

Screening for sleep apnea and studying the use of postoperative CPAP in sleep apnea patients: A narrative review

Joel Maruthanal[1], MD, MPH
Autumn Forde[1], BA
Akanksha Arora[1], BS
Michael Heustess McLatchey[1], BA
Tolulope Oladimeji[2], MD, MPH
and Emmanuel O Keku[1], MD, MA, MSPH
[1]Department of Public Health and Preventive Medicine, St George's University, School of Medicine, St George, Grenada, West Indies
[2]Department of Pathophysiology, St George's University, School of Medicine, St George, Grenada, West Indies

Abstract

Sleep apnea is an underdiagnosed condition that plagues many individuals in the United States of America. In terms of surgery, sleep apnea is a comorbidity that may lead to postoperative complications. Various methods have been used to decrease postoperative complications. One such application is the use of continuous positive airway pressure (CPAP). The aim of this study was to provide information on whether secondary prevention (via questionnaire screenings) and tertiary prevention (via postoperative CPAP administration in all sleep apnea patients) could lead to better health outcomes. In this study, the researcher conducted computer searches of the Cochrane library, PubMed and Science Direct databases. The medical

In: Public Health
Editors: Emmanuel O Keku and Joav Merrick
ISBN: 979-8-89113-083-8

subject headings (MeSH) keywords were sleep apnea syndromes and CPAP, and general surgery or preoperative care or postoperative care or postoperative complications or length of stay. English language articles from 2009 onwards were selected for review. Inclusion and exclusion criteria addressed which articles were selected for this narrative review. Review of the literature yielded 86 results. This was further narrowed down to 28 results. They were then analyzed into the following categories: CPAP use, preoperative care, postoperative care, postoperative complications and length of stay. In conclusion, sleep apnea should be screened for in all preoperative patients and CPAP should be used more in the postoperative setting.

Keywords: sleep apnea, continuous positive airway pressure, preoperative care, postoperative care, and postoperative complications

Introduction

Sleep apnea is a prevalent condition in the world (1). Estimates report nearly one billion people have obstructive sleep apnea (2). In the United States (US) alone, it is estimated that 22 million Americans have sleep apnea and 80% of them do not know they have it (1). Sleep apnea can lead to consequences such as hypertension, cardiovascular issues, cerebrovascular issues and even death (3). Luckily, it can be diagnosed and treatments (surgical and non-surgical) exist. Several questionnaires (STOPBANG, Berlin, Epworth Sleepiness Scale) are used for early detection (4, 5).

Some non-surgical treatments involve weight loss, CPAP use, oral and nasal appliances, and limited use of medicine (6). In the surgical setting, sleep apnea has been associated with increased morbidity and mortality (7, 8). Postoperatively, sleep apnea patients are more at risk for complications such as hypoxia, cardiac and respiratory events, and prolonged hospital stay (5, 7, 8). Since sleep apnea has been identified as a comorbidity for postoperative complications, protocols/suggestions have been developed (9, 10). Some protocols try to identify sleep apnea patients before surgery and suggest using CPAP after surgery (9-11).

The aim of this study was to present information about diagnosing sleep apnea preoperatively and using CPAP postoperatively, as secondary, and tertiary prevention respectively. If sleep apnea is added to preoperative evaluations, CPAP or other methods will be used postoperatively and complications in sleep apnea patients could be reduced. As sleep apnea is prevalent and underdiagnosed, screenings and CPAP use would lead to better outcomes for both patients and hospitals (12, 13).

Methods

This narrative review followed the following five steps: 1. Identifying the research question; 2. Search methods for identifying relevant studies; 3. Study selection; 4. Charting the data, collating, and summarizing; 5. Reporting the results.

Identify the research question

Will CPAP use in the postoperative setting reduce complications in sleep apnea patients as a form of tertiary prevention? Should sleep apnea evaluation be used in the preoperative setting as secondary prevention?

Search methods for identifying relevant studies

In this study, computer searches of the Cochrane Library, PubMed and Science Direct databases were conducted. The medical subject headings (MeSH) keywords were sleep apnea syndromes, CPAP, general surgery, preoperative care, postoperative complications and length of stay. Articles from 2009 onwards were selected for review. Inclusion and exclusion criteria addressed which articles were selected for this narrative review.

Study selection

Using the above MeSH terms, an initial search yielded a list of papers. After reviewing the titles and abstracts of these papers, we included the relevant articles based on my inclusion and exclusion criteria. After reviewing the articles, we used the included articles to form an overall narrative on preventative measures for sleep apnea patients who will undergo surgery and a narrative on postoperative care.

Inclusion criteria

Papers involving the diagnosis of sleep apnea, and CPAP use in perioperative sleep apnea patients were included. English language articles from 2009 onwards were selected. Papers revolving around postoperative complications, such as oxygen desaturation, cardiac events, respiratory events, and increased length of stay, were also included.

Exclusion criteria

Excluded papers included those about procedures to treat sleep apnea, those about postoperative complications in non-sleep apnea patients, and those focusing primarily on obesity.

Charting the data, collating and summarizing

Data was summarized in Figure 1 and Table 1.

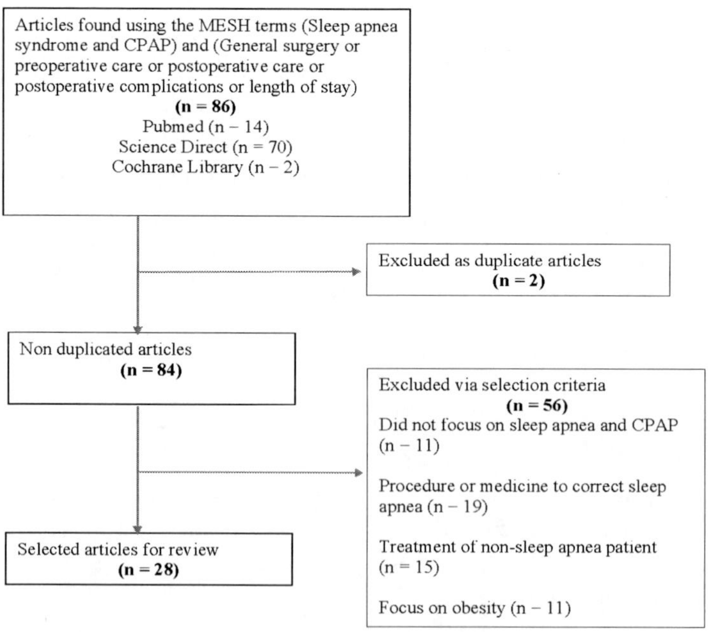

Figure 1. Article selection process.

Table 1. Sleep apnea in relation to several categories

Category	Number of articles	Results	Overall narrative
CPAP use	6	All six articles discussed how postoperative CPAP use was beneficial in outcomes in sleep apnea patients. Two of the six also recommend preoperative CPAP use.	CPAP should be used both before and after surgery in sleep apnea patients
Preoperative setting	8	Eight articles discussed the importance of screening for sleep apnea minimize the risks. Some went into further detail as to how different factors play a role in preoperative evaluation. One article goes on to say polysomnography should be routine preoperative screening in the bariatric population.	Questionnaires such as STOP BANG should be standard in preoperative screening for all patients. While polysomnography is the gold standard of diagnosis, screening should be done first.
Postoperative care	4	Postoperative care varies from place to place. These four articles discussed the importance of monitoring postoperative patients who have sleep apnea and the importance of CPAP use.	More focus should be done on proactive monitoring and CPAP use in the postoperative setting. Less complications will occur if we are proactive instead of reactive.
Postoperative complications	7	Five articles discussed how sleep apnea patients tended to have more postoperative complications and how being treated with CPAP alleviated/prevented some complications. On the other hand, 2 articles did not find major adverse outcomes or clear associations between OSA and negative outcomes. However, both papers suggest further study.	While most of the papers discussed how sleep apnea leads to increased risk of postoperative complications, some papers did not agree. It would be prudent to have further studies.
Length of stay	3	One article described decreased length of stay in patients who received perioperative CPAP. The other two articles reported sleep apnea patients tend to have increased lengths of stay.	Perioperative CPAP use should decrease length of stay in postoperative patients with sleep apnea

Reporting the findings

Results were discussed in the following categories: CPAP use, preoperative care, postoperative care, postoperative complications and length of stay. Each category was in reference to sleep apnea. Each category discussed how their interactions affected sleep apnea patients, how many articles support a link between the category and sleep apnea, and what overall narrative there was for that category.

Results

For all databases, the following search term was used: (CPAP and sleep apnea) and (general surgery or preoperative care or postoperative care or postoperative complications or length of stay or general surgery). The Cochrane Library Database yielded two results. The PubMed database yielded 14 results and lastly, Science Direct yielded 70 results. Figure 1 illustrates the selection process among these 86 results. Ultimately, 28 articles were selected for this review. Table 1 illustrates how the selected papers contributed to this review.

Discussion

In general, most articles supported preoperative screening for sleep apnea and CPAP use in the postoperative setting for sleep apnea patients.

CPAP use

CPAP has been used in sleep apnea patients for many years. It prevents narrowing of the airway. Although it is a mainstay in the treatment of sleep apnea, adherence is a problem (14, 15). In general, it seems that patients do not like using the CPAP machine. This is understandable as having a large mask on one's face that blows air into one's throat can be uncomfortable. Additionally, some machines are better than others. Some might have better humidifiers so dry throats and noses are not a problem. Others have more advanced technology, and they don't make as much noise. Atkins and Fleisher

(14) also discussed the importance of CPAP-BiPAP in the postoperative setting. Other articles recommend the use of CPAP both before and after surgery (16, 17). Though CPAP use should not lead one to develop a lax attitude. Hillman and Eastwood (18) noted the importance of CPAP, but they stressed the importance of good monitoring. Ramachandran (19) also noted that CPAP was one among many factors that leads to reduced risk. Thus, these papers suggested CPAP use is beneficial in the postoperative setting for patients who have sleep apnea. Further evidence of the importance of CPAP can be seen in the other categories of this narrative review.

Preoperative care

Preoperative care consists of several exams that may vary depending on the patient and surgery. Some typical examinations may include chest X-ray, electrocardiogram, blood tests and urinalysis. Other tests may be ordered as well. In the case of surgical patients, it is imperative that screening be done to minimize risk as many are not diagnosed with sleep apnea (20-23). As mentioned earlier, several questionnaires have been developed. One simple and effective screening tool is the STOP-BANG questionnaire (24). By screening for sleep apnea, there can be more preparation for "effective perioperative management" (25). In addition, it is important to look at other factors such as suspicion of OSA, type of surgery, anticipation of pain medications, availability of emergency airways and respiratory equipment in the preoperative evaluation (26). Lastly, one article also discussed using routine polysomnography in the bariatric population (27). Although polysomnography is the gold standard of diagnosing sleep apnea, it might not be feasible for everyone to undergo the test.

After reviewing these articles, we believe that preoperative screening with questionnaires should become standard protocol. This form of secondary prevention would be quite simple to do. In the event of a positive screening, a patient may be given better care as more risks can be accounted for.

Postoperative care

Postoperative care also varies among patients and surgeries. However, one commonality in all postoperative care is the importance of monitoring. Even though the surgical procedure was done, complications can occur. Vigilant monitoring can catch small problems before they become large complications. Ramachandran et al. (28) demonstrated this through their pilot study of alerting respiratory therapists. In their study, they let respiratory therapists receive alerts about patients with sleep apnea or risk factors for sleep apnea. Thus, someone was ready to start monitoring the postoperative patient. After the 5-month duration of the study, it was found that no acute respiratory compromise events occurred. While this is only one study, that was quite impressive.

Another article also demonstrated the variations of postoperative care. Tong et al. (29) noted that some healthcare workers did not accept noninvasive positive pressure ventilation (NIPPV) due to possible complications of anastomotic dehiscence in obese bariatric surgery. In their review, they went on to show that there was not an increased rate of anastomotic dehiscence in patients who received NIPPV. Another article reported that along with sleep apnea patients, all patients who screened positive for sleep apnea should receive consideration for CPAP postoperatively (30). It shows that there are guidelines and suggestions, but no firm protocol. Nevertheless, thinking should not be discouraged. This can be seen in the last article of this section. When it comes to discharging or monitoring, several factors should be looked at. Seet et al. (31) discussed three main focuses of postoperative disposition. They are invasiveness of surgery, severity of sleep apnea, and requirements of opioids. Based on these factors, a patient may be discharged home, stay for monitoring, or remain in the surgical ward. Generally, there seems to be leeway in the use of CPAP in the postoperative setting. But if anything is to be inferred from the articles in this category, it is that CPAP is useful in the postoperative setting and that vigilance is crucial.

Postoperative Complications

Postoperative complications can be a result of various factors. In addition, there are many types of postoperative complications. Only this category had differing opinions. In a small study by Alexa et al. (32) major adverse outcomes were not found in primary central sleep apnea patients who underwent procedures that required anesthesia. In a second study, De Raaff et al. (33) noted that there was no clear association between obstructive sleep apnea and “cardiopulmonary morbidity, ICU admissions, mortality, and length of stay.” However, in this study it must be noted that some patients may have been optimized with CPAP therapy.

On the other hand, several articles have found that sleep apnea patients tend to have more risk of postoperative complications. Nagappa et al. (34) reports that patients who had OSA had higher odds of experiencing major adverse cardiac or cerebrovascular events (33% higher odds) or postoperative atrial fibrillation (18% higher odds). Suen et al. (35) agreed that sleep apnea patients have increased risk of postoperative complications, but they specified that complications seem to scale with sleep apnea severity. Subramani et al. (36) also noted postoperative complications including death and near miss events. Lastly, Lam et al. (37) discussed how there have been associations between sleep disordered breathing and postoperative delirium.

In a randomized clinical trial (38) patients who received auto titrated CPAP (APAP) had "significantly reduced postoperative AHI and improved saturation." Hence, CPAP should be used in the postoperative setting.

Length of stay

Length of stay is constantly under scrutiny at various levels. Hospital administrators and healthcare workers worry about longer lengths of stay, which lead to poorer health outcomes and more financial burden. Additionally, most patients do not wish to remain in a hospital/medical setting. In terms of sleep apnea, it has been reported that sleep apnea patients tend to have increased length of stay (38, 39). Additionally, in a randomized control study, Melesse et al. (40) demonstrated that perioperative CPAP use decreased length of hospital stay among a variety of other benefits.

Limitations

Some limitations of this paper included restricting the search to only English literature and using only three databases for literature review.

Conclusion

Review of these articles demonstrated that pre-operative screening for sleep apnea and post-operative treatment of CPAP for sleep apnea surgery patients are beneficial and should be incorporated into normal protocol. As previously thought, sleep apnea is still underdiagnosed. However, it seems that more emphasis is being put for diagnosing and treating sleep apnea. Secondly, while there are many factors that play a role in postoperative complications, CPAP use in sleep apnea patients tend to reduce some of these complications. In terms of public health, this secondary and tertiary prevention will yield better health outcomes.

Recommendation

Sleep apnea questionnaires should be given to all patients (that are not already diagnosed with sleep apnea) prior to surgical procedures. Additionally, there should be more standard protocols for CPAP use in sleep apnea patients in the postoperative setting. Postoperative sleep apnea patients should use CPAP. Finally, it would be beneficial to have further studies to show the benefits of both screening for sleep apnea and the use of CPAP in the postoperative setting.

References

[1] American Sleep Apnea Association. Sleep apnea information for clinicians. URL: https://www.sleepapnea.org/learn/sleep-apnea-information-clinicians/.

[2] Benjafield AV, Ayas NT, Eastwood PR, Heinzer R, Ip MSM, Morrell. MJ, et al. Estimation of the global prevalence and burden of obstructive sleep apnea: A literature-based analysis. Lancet Respir Med 2019;7(8):687–98.

[3] Javaheri S, Barbe F, Campos-Rodriguez F, Dempsey JA, Khayat R, Javaheri S, et al. Sleep apnea. J Am Coll Cardiol 2017;69(7): 841–58.

[4] Chiu HY, Chen PY, Chuang LP, Chen NH, Tu YK, Hsieh YJ, et al. Diagnostic accuracy of the Berlin questionnaire, STOP-BANG, STOP, and Epworth sleepiness scale in detecting obstructive sleep apnea: A bivariate meta-analysis. Sleep Med Rev 2017;36:57–70.

[5] Proczko MA, Stepaniak PS, Quelerij MD, Lely FHVD, Smulders J, Kaska L, et al. STOP-Bang and the effect on patient outcome and length of hospital stay when patients are not using continuous positive airway pressure. J Anesth 2014;28(6): 891–7.

[6] Semelka M, Wilson J, Floyd R. Diagnosis, and treatment of obstructive sleep apnea in adults. Am Fam Physician 2016;94(5):355–60.

[7] Mador MJ, Goplani S, Gottumukkala VA, El-Solh AA, Akashdeep K, Khadka G, Abo-Khamis M. Postoperative complications in obstructive sleep apnea. Sleep Breath 2012;17(2):727–34.

[8] Liao P, Yegneswaran B, Vairavanathan S, Zilberman P, Chung F. Postoperative complications in patients with obstructive sleep apnea: A retrospective matched cohort study. Can J Anaesth 2009;56(11):819–28.
[9] Mickelson SA. Anesthetic and postoperative management of the obstructive sleep apnea patient. Oral Maxillofac Surg Clin North Am 2009;21(4):425–34.
[10] Qassamali SR, Lagoo-Deenadayalan S, Mcdonald S, Morgan B, Goode V. The importance of the STOP- BANG questionnaire as a preoperative assessment tool for the elderly population. Geriatr Nurs 2019;40(5):536–9.
[11] Wolfe RM, Pomerantz J, Miller DE, Weiss-Coleman R, Solomonides T. Obstructive sleep apnea: Preoperative screening and postoperative care. J Am Board Fam Med 2016;29(2):263–75.
[12] Hillman DR, Jungquist CR, Auckley D. Perioperative implementation of noninvasive positive airway pressure therapies. Respir Care 2018;63(4):479–87.
[13] Liao P, Luo Q, Elsaid H, Kang W, Shapiro CM, Chung F. Perioperative auto-titrated continuous positive airway pressure treatment in surgical patients with obstructive sleep apnea. Anesthesiology 2013;119(4):837–47.
[14] Atkins JH, Fleisher LA. Value from the patients' and payers' perspectives. Anesthesiol Clin 2015;33(4):651–8.
[15] Sundar E, Malhotra A. Unanswered questions in sleep and anesthesia. Sleep Med Clin 2013;8(1):165–75.
[16] Chung F, Nagappa M, Singh M, Mokhlesi B. CPAP in the perioperative setting. Chest 2016;149(2):586–97.
[17] Taylor A, Deboard Z, Gauvin JM. Prevention of postoperative pulmonary complications. Surg Clin North Am 2015;95(2):237–54.
[18] Hillman DR, Eastwood PR. Upper airway, obstructive sleep apnea, and anesthesia. Sleep Med Clin 2013;8(1):23–8.
[19] Ramachandran SK. Obstructive sleep apnea and perioperative complications. Sleep Med Clin 2013;8(1):93–103.
[20] Tamisier R, Fabre F, Odonoghue F, Lévy P, Payen JF, Pépin JL. Anesthesia and sleep apnea. Sleep Med Rev 2018;40:79–92.
[21] Raveendran R, Wong J, Chung F. Morbid obesity, sleep apnea, obesity hypoventilation syndrome: Are we sleepwalking into disaster? Perioper Care Oper Room Manag 2017; 9:24–32.
[22] Veenstra A, Untalan E. Implications and interventions related to obstructive sleep apnea. Crit Care Nurs Clin North Am 2014;26(4):499–509.
[23] Gay PC. Positive airway pressure therapy for perioperative patients. Sleep Med Clin 2013:8(1):121–8.
[24] Wood KL, Besecker BY. Perioperative issues and sleep-disordered breathing. Crit Care Clin 2015;31(3):497–510.
[25] Subramani Y, Wong J, Nagappa M, Chung F. The benefits of perioperative screening for sleep apnea in surgical patients. Sleep Med Clin 2017;12(1):123–35.
[26] Kaw R. Perioperative complications in patients with obstructive sleep apnea. Sleep Med Clin 2013;8(1):129–34.
[27] Bohman JK, Kor DJ. Advances in perioperative pulmonary protection strategies. Adv Anesth 2014;32(1):89–117.

[28] Ramachandran SK, Kheterpal S, Haas CF, Saran KA, Tremper KK. Automated notification of suspected obstructive sleep apnea patients to the perioperative respiratory therapist: a pilot study. Respir Care 2010;55(4):414–8.

[29] Tong S, Gower J, Morgan A, Gadbois K, Wisbach G. Noninvasive positive pressure ventilation in the immediate post–bariatric surgery care of patients with obstructive sleep apnea: a systematic review. Surg Obes Relat Dis 2017; 13(7): 1227–33.

[30] Brabeck DM, Brabeck MC. Controversies in perioperative medicine. Hosp Med Clin 2017;6(2):163–75.

[31] Seet E, Han TL, Chung F. Perioperative clinical pathways to manage sleep-disordered breathing. Sleep Med Clin 2013;8(1):105–20.

[32] Alexa A, Mansukhani MP, Gali B, Deljou A, Sprung J, Weingarten TN. Primary central sleep apnea and anesthesia: A retrospective case series. Can J Anaesth 2018;65(8):884–92.

[33] de Raaff CA, Coblijn UK, de Vries N, van Wagensveld BA. Is fear for postoperative cardiopulmonary complications after bariatric surgery in patients with obstructive sleep apnea justified? A systematic review. Am J Surg 2016;211(4):793-801.

[34] Nagappa M, Ho G, Patra J, Wong J, Singh M, Kaw R, et. al. Postoperative outcomes in obstructive sleep apnea patients undergoing cardiac surgery. Anesth Analg 2017;125(6):2030–7.

[35] Suen C, Ryan CM, Mubashir T, Ayas NT, Abrahamyan L, Wong J, Chung F. Sleep study and oximetry parameters for predicting postoperative complications in patients with OSA. Chest 2017;155(4):855–67.

[36] Subramani Y, Nagappa M, Wong J, Patra J, Chung F. Death or near-death in patients with obstructive sleep apnoea: A compendium of case reports of critical complications. Br J Anaesth 2017;119(5):885–99.

[37] Lam EWK, Chung F, Wong J. Sleep-disordered breathing, postoperative delirium, and cognitive impairment. Anesth Analg 2017;124(5):1626–35.

[38] Hillman DR, Platt PR, Eastwood PR. Anesthesia, sleep, and upper airway collapsibility. Anesthesiol Clin 2010;28(3):443–55.

[39] De Raaff CAL, Gorter-Stam MAW, de Vries N, Sinha AC, Bonjer HJ, Chung F, et al. Peri-operative management of obstructive sleep apnea in bariatric surgery: A consensus guideline. Surg Obes Relat Dis 2017;13(7):1095-109.

[40] Melesse DY, Mekonnen ZA, Kassahun HG, Chekol WB. Evidence based perioperative optimization of patients with obstructive sleep apnea in resource limited areas: A systematic review. Int J Surg Open 2020; 23:23–4.

Chapter 6

How complementary therapies and aerobic exercises influence cancer

David A Patch[1], MD, MEd
Samantha Bhambrah[1], BS
Samuel Ianuario[1], BS
Anthony Whyte[1], BS
Divya Situt[1], BS
Tolulope Oladimeji[2], MD, MPH
and Emmanuel O Keku[1], MD, MA, MSPH
[1]Department of Public Health and Preventive Medicine, St George's University, School of Medicine, St George, Grenada, West Indies
[2]Department of Pathophysiology, St George's University, School of Medicine, St George, Grenada, West Indies

Abstract

This literature review examined the positive effects (e.g., cardiovascular endurance, strength, reduction of stress) of aerobic exercise combined with complementary therapies on cancer survival rates. The literature suggests that complementary therapies and aerobic exercise may serve as an effective alternative treatment in decreasing cancer-related fatigue, improving immune system function, and increasing quality of life in cancer patients. Numerous research investigations reported positive correlations between complementary therapies and their role in suppressing adverse effects of conventional treatments such as cachexia, cancer-related fatigue, and negative emotions. However, dosage guidelines for these alternative treatments are lacking and concern about

In: Public Health
Editors: Emmanuel O Keku and Joav Merrick
ISBN: 979-8-89113-083-8

the side effects and interactions between complementary modalities and conventional treatments remain. Additionally, the review suggested complementary therapies such as tai chi, yoga, acupuncture, and meditation may enhance the effects of conventional medical treatments. Further studies are warranted to understand the underlying mechanisms responsible for the effects of these therapies in cancer patient populations.

Keywords: cancer, complementary therapies, aerobic exercise, survival

Introduction

In the United States (US) today, almost nine million people have a history of cancer (1). The majority are survivors, however approximately four million people are living with cancer (1). According to Young-McCaughan et al. (1) cancer is in general a fatal disease and for most forms of epithelial cancers there tends to be an exponential increasing relationship between age and cancer incidence or mortality. Thus, age is the single most important determinant for risk of cancer, and after cardiovascular diseases, cancer is the most common cause of death in many countries (1).

Some advances in cancer treatment for certain cancers have occurred during the last decades; however, this seems only to have improved cancer mortality among children, young and middle-aged persons (1). The proportion of people over the age of 65 years has increased from around 5% to over 20% in some Western European countries during the last few decades and it is estimated that in the next century around 25% of the population in many countries will be older than 65 years (1). These trends have incentivized cancer survivors to alter their dietary and physical activity regimens using complementary and alternative medicine (CAM) (2). The growing interest in CAM among cancer survivors is the driving force behind further research concerning the relationship between complementary therapies, aerobic exercise, and cancer survivorship (2).

Complementary therapies can be defined as a group of diverse medical practices, products, and techniques that are not recognized as conventional medicine (2). General complementary therapies used as supportive measures in conjunction with mainstream cancer care include alternative medicines, mind-body techniques, energy and biological based therapies, and manipulative body treatments (2). Specific types of complementary therapies include herbs and vitamins, spiritual healing, massage, acupuncture, relaxation, lifestyles, and special diets (2). According to Anderson et al. (2), 64% of the US cancer patient populations have used at least one type of CAM modality during the course of their cancer treatment plan. Complementary therapies are utilized by cancer patients to enhance the benefits of conventional treatments such as radiation, and chemotherapy. The use of CAM has been shown to be specifically effective in cancer patients who are undergoing multiple treatments, concomitant diseases, and other treatment-related symptoms (2).

Prevalence of complementary therapies

National surveys of the general population have found an increase in the use of complementary therapies, and alternative medicine, around the world (2). One such study conducted in the United States between 1990, and 1997, observed an increase in complementary use from 33.8% to 42.1% among cancer patients (3). However, it is important to note that the research indicates that the effects of herbal medication may result in unfavorable side effects (2). The use of herbal medications, and high-dose antioxidants, may induce negative interactions between physician prescribed drugs, radiation therapy, and chemotherapeutic agents (2). This constitutes the primary reason for why most oncologists discourage their patients from experimenting with these types of therapies during treatment. More scientific research is warranted on the use of complementary therapies in relation to their dosage, frequency of use, and side effects. This in turn, will allow health care professions to administer safe recommendations based on empirical evidence supporting the use of CAM.

The effects of lifestyle on cancer

To better understand the effects of complementary therapies and their influence upon cancer, researchers have conducted studies to examine the role of lifestyle modifications such as diet, and activity levels, that are associated with reduced risk of recurrence of breast cancer. A prospective study conducted was designed using 1,490 women diagnosed, and treated, for stage I breast cancer between 1991 and 2000 (4). The researchers found there was a

50% increase in the likelihood of cancer survivorship among those participants who consumed five, or more, servings of fruits and vegetables daily: in addition to exercising six days a week for 30 minutes. Furthermore, a study investigated the effects of isoflavone consumption in 5,042 Chinese breast cancer survivors and found that Asian women who ingested the highest concentration of soy foods had the least recurrence of breast cancer, and an increased life expectancy (5). Similarly, another investigation found that postmenopausal American women, who took Tamoxifen and ingested the equivalent of isoflavones consumed in an Asian diet, demonstrated a 60% reduction in breast cancer recurrence (6). However, due to differences in the epigenetics of American breast cancer survivors in comparison to Asian breast cancer survivors, the consumption of soy foods equaling the equivalent of the Asian diet warrants more research currently (5).

One of the mainstream treatment options for cancer patients is chemotherapy. However, recent research has indicated that although chemotherapy improves survival rates it also induces harmful toxicity to healthy tissues by producing reactive oxygen species (ROS) (7). As a result of chemotherapy lowering the body's natural physiological defense mechanisms, cancer patients are at an increased risk of experiencing oxidative stress and free-radical formation. Regarding prostate cancer, the use of vitamins, minerals, herbs, vitamin E, and lycopene are thought to specifically protect the prostate (8). Even though there is an increased interest in the use of CAM, it is still a relatively low topic between doctor and patient.

High-dose antioxidant therapy and cancer

Antioxidants serve to defend healthy cells from free radicals and prevent uncontrollable cellular proliferation (7). The effects of vitamins C and E on antioxidant status have been shown to exhibit protective effects against damage caused by both radiation, and chemotherapy (7). In addition, vitamin E has been hypothesized to augment antineoplastic activity through suppressing the peroxidation of lipids (7). According to Suhail et al. (7), vitamin E and C are recognized as the most essential naturally occurring antioxidant vitamins and may be supportive in ameliorating oxidative stress generated during cancer reducing therapies such as chemotherapy, and radiation. It has been proposed that the antioxidant effect of vitamin C derives from its ability to lose a hydrogen atom and to form a reasonably stable ascorbate free radical (7). Additionally, the co-administration of vitamin C and

E has been found to work synergistically in restoring the antioxidant status and reducing DNA damage in breast-cancer patients undergoing chemotherapy (7). Moreover, vitamin supplementation in breast cancer patients may also function to reduce the side effects commonly associated with conventional treatments.

Diet and supplements should be included under complementary practices used to enhance the effects of conventional treatments (2). High-dose antioxidant therapies usually ameliorate the symptoms caused by cancer rather than harm cancer patients (7). Antioxidants are recognized by their ability to regulate free radicals and reduce the formation of mutations (7). A study showed that in large concentrations, intravenous vitamin C produces levels of hydrogen peroxide in the cells that have the capacity to function as a mild and nontoxic form of chemotherapy (9). Further investigations have shown that various amounts and types of antioxidants can counteract nutritional deficiencies, disorganize the life cycle of cancer cells, and induce apoptosis (7). Antioxidants have also been shown to suppress the side effects of chemotherapy, regulate inflammation, ease pain, inhibit the production of free radicals, improve quality of life and appetite, and may extend life expectancy (9). The implementation of high-dose antioxidants therapies in cancerous populations may provide benefits by supporting a complex series of biochemical pathways and gene-regulating activities (9). In addition to the effects of dietary modifications in cancer patient populations, complementary therapies such as tai chi, yoga, breathing, acupuncture, and mindfulness have been investigated as well.

Mind-body movement therapy

Aromatase inhibitors are a standard treatment for postmenopausal women coping with hormone-receptor positive breast cancer because the drug inhibits the conversion of testosterone to estrogen (10). However, aromatase-inhibitor associated arthralgia (AIAA) is a major side effect experienced by breast cancer survivors (10). The mechanism by which aromatase inhibitors express their effects is unknown, however; research indicates that suppressed estrogens levels can cause bone loss and disrupt bone remodeling and resorption (11). According to Galantino et al. (10), the majority of breast cancer survivor's experience arthralgia during conventional treatment; yet very few interventions have been implemented to target this side effect. As a result of approximately 354.2 million complementary visits made by US adults in 2007, studies examining symptom management for cancer survivors continue to grow (2).

Tai chi serves as a weight-bearing, mind-body movement therapy that has been shown to improve balance, strength, and bone formation with a decrease in bone resorption in cancer survivors (12). The premise of tai chi is founded upon helping an individual become healthier by focusing on deep breathing, slow movement patterns, and total body awareness. A study examined the impact a tai chi intervention had on breast cancer patients, and it was found that tai chi was effective in reducing stress, anxiety, depression, cancer-related fatigue, and improving emotional well-being (10). Mind-body movement therapies used in breast cancer survivors have been shown to reduce treatment-related side effects of conventional treatment such as inflammatory responses and other biomarkers (13). As seen in physical activity, tai chi also increases the number of endorphins in the brain and neuropsychological health (14).

Additionally, researchers have reported that tai chi reduces stress and anxiety in breast cancer patients through mindfulness, movement, and breathing exercises, which have been found to reduce joint pain (15). Regarding the mind-body relationship, tai chi encourages both awareness and proprioception (10). Hence, tai chi has been thought to serve as an ideal therapy to improve dynamic stabilization, whole body coordination, and flexibility. Thus, the research indicates that the use of tai chi can suppress the side effects of aromatase inhibitor-associated arthralgias (AIAA) and improve overall quality of life in breast cancer patients (10).

Cancer is often associated with sleep disturbance, stress, anxiety, chronic fatigue, and decreased quality of life (16). Despite numerous advancements in the evolution of conventional cancer treatment options, effective symptom management interventions warrant more attention (16). The regulation and expansion of breath can serve as an effective therapy to reduce oxidative stress and provide health benefits (16). Research also indicates that breathing exercises may help induce a relaxed state by enhancing the body's parasympathetic tone (17). Additionally, a study conducted by Dhruva et al. (16) investigated the effects of yoga breathing techniques among 44 female breast cancer patients undergoing chemotherapy over a 10-week period. The researchers found that patients who performed 3.2 hours of yoga practice per week experienced significant improvements in sleep disturbance, anxiety, quality of life, and cancer chemotherapy associated symptoms (16). Therefore, the results of this study indicate that the breathing techniques performed in yoga interventions may pose health benefits among women breast cancer patients undergoing chemotherapy. However, further research is warranted to determine the exact nature of the underlying mechanisms by which these benefits may occur.

Some studies indicate that up to 30% of breast cancer patients will develop psychologic morbidity within 1 year of diagnosis (18). Meanwhile, yoga interventions have attracted the interest of researchers for their potential therapeutic applications in breast cancer patients (19). According to Zhang et al. (19), randomized controlled trials have demonstrated that yoga-based interventions reduce cancer-related fatigue, depression, anxiety, and chemotherapy related side effects. A meta-analysis used to examine the effects of yoga on psychologic function, and quality of life, found that yoga induced changes in breath volume, decreased heart rate, and reduced negative emotions (19). However, the authors concluded that further research is warranted to understand the direct effects of yoga-based interventions before clinicians can advocate yoga as a routine treatment option for breast cancer patients. In addition, the effects of yoga symptom management in cancer patients, acupuncture has gained popularity for its role in ameliorating disease related symptoms.

Role of acupuncture in cancer patients

Acupuncture has been found to function as an effective treatment option for managing the side effects induced by chemotherapy and radiation during cancer therapy (20). According to Jaung-Geng and Yi-Hung (20), the two strategies most used to perform acupuncture consist of manual acupuncture (MA), and electroacupuncture (EA). Neuropathic pain has been documented as the most difficult type of pain to treat in cancer patients because of its unwillingness to respond well to conventional cancer treatments (21).

Another complication commonly found in patients undergoing radiation therapy for head and neck cancer is xerostomia, or dry mouth (20). This condition is caused by the toxic exposure of radiation to the salivary glands. According to Jaung-Geng and Yi-Hung (20), the reduction in salivary flow is dependent upon the radiation dose and the surface area of the damaged salivary glands. A recent study examined the impact of acupuncture treatments on patients with head and neck cancer (22). The researchers reported that patients who received acupuncture showed improved salivary flow rates, and ameliorated xerostomia-related symptoms such as difficulty masticating, swallowing, and speaking clearly (22). Acupuncture has also been observed to relieve chemotherapy induced nausea and vomiting, in addition to sedative effects (20). The culmination of the proposed effects of acupuncture suggests that it may serve as an effective therapy for cancer patients looking to manage their symptoms. As with acupuncture, the effects of mindfulness based cognitive therapy (MBCT) in cancer patient populations have also gained much attention.

Mindfulness based cognitive therapy

Men with advanced prostate cancer are subject to additional challenges in comparison to men with localized disease; in addition, men with advanced prostate have reported higher levels of psychological distress and higher rates of depression (23). Therefore, Chambers et al. (23) conducted a study to examine the effects of MBCT. The practice of mindfulness in cancer patients has been said to open awareness, control negative emotions, and improve positive thought (23). Due to cancer patients commonly reporting poor states of mind, MBCT has been reported to induce positive changes in acceptance, self-control, personal growth, and self-regulation in patients with prostate cancer (23).

The emotion regulation strategies exercised in mindfulness meditation-based stress reduction (MBSR) have also been shown to help cancer patients prevent worrying about the future, living in fear, and being in a constant state of denial. Using MBSR, a study assessed its impact on mood disturbance, and stress symptoms, during a 7-week program consisting of 89 patients with a variety of cancer diagnoses (24). The researchers found that patients who completed the program experienced improvements of 65% on mood and 35% on stress symptoms compared to the control group (24). Patients reported less of a decrease in tension, depression, anger, central neurologic symptoms, gastrointestinal symptoms, and concentration problems following the MBSR intervention. It is also important to note the women in the MBSR group reported greater improvements in overall disease-related symptoms in comparison to men. However, further research is warranted to understand the underlying mechanism for this finding. In addition to mindfulness, the effects of aerobic exercise have also been subject to investigation in exploration of their potential influence on cancer. The research suggests physical activity can serve as an effective activity to alleviate the adverse effects of cancer related symptoms, side effects, and conventional treatments (25).

Mechanism of aerobic exercise in cancer patients

Exercise can counteract some of the symptoms caused by cancer and some of the adverse effects associated with treatment, including body weight fluctuations, loss of muscle mass, nausea, vomiting, difficulties eating or digesting food, mood changes, fatigue, and other psychological disturbances (26). Cancer or its treatment may require low physical activity from the patient, which can result in reduced fitness, endurance, and muscle strength that exercise could ameliorate later (26). In addition, there is growing interest in the role exercise may play in preventing cancer recurrence and improving long-term survival (26). However, cancer-related fatigue must be considered in relation to cancer survivors' capacity to engage in regular exercise bouts.

Cancer-related fatigue reportedly affects 70% to 100% of people with cancer, occurring for the duration of treatment or after completion (27). The ultimate cause of cancer-related fatigue is largely unknown, though factors contributing to it have been suggested. If no potentially causative factor can be identified, the guidelines suggest a variety of possible approaches to revive vitality. One of the notable non-pharmacological approaches is to increase activity, which has shown to possibly reduce both the physical effects and the psychological stress associated with cancer treatments, improve mood, and reduce anxiety and fear in patients (27). The impact of physical activity in decreasing the risk of breast cancer recurrence continues to be studied (25). Recently, the American College of Sports Medicine (ACSM) published consensus derived guidelines for exercise for people surviving cancer, which stated that exercise is safe and results in improved physical functioning, quality of life and reduced fatigue (27).

Studies have shown that women with breast cancer that were less active reported higher fatigue (28). Furthermore, physical exercise improves overall health and enhances mood and quality of life (QOL), which can be defined as overall pleasure, comfort, and enjoyment in one's life. Wu and others (28) designed a rehabilitation program consisting of a walking program and a support group for patients with breast cancer receiving chemotherapy. The participants demonstrated an improvement in physical functioning, with a decrease in fatigue and emotional distress (28). Improved physical functioning and less fatigue, anxiety, and difficulty sleeping also were reported by those who participated in a walking program during the radiation treatment (28). As a result, the use of physical exercise programs in cancer patient populations has gained the attention of researchers.

Participation in a structured exercise program can provide patients with a safe environment in which to exercise at intensities appropriate to their individual needs. Exercise prescription in patients with cancer is an aspect of cancer rehabilitation that demands the expertise of a multidisciplinary team that includes oncology nurses, exercise physiologists, physical therapists, oncology physicians, and people with cancer (1). Physical exercise programs offered during, as well as following, cancer treatment is becoming more common in the usual care of patients with cancer (1). In general, the guidelines recommend that all exercise programs should be individualized; taking into consideration treatments received and associated symptoms, comorbidities, contraindications to activity, and patient prognosis.

Impact of therapy exercise on cancer patients

Exercise self-efficacy (ESE) is defined as the self-assessed motivation of respondents to exercise regularly given their personal, situational and social impediments (29). Exercise outcome expectations include positive or negative physical effects as well as psychosocial effects of exercise (29). Specifically, patients with breast cancer who performed a moderate level of aerobic exercise during adjuvant cancer treatment experienced less intense nausea at treatment completion (29). A moderate level of aerobic exercise is recommended during adjuvant cancer treatment considering its possibility to support a decline in nausea intensity as well as the benefits of alleviating other symptoms from adjuvant cancer treatment. The results of one study showed that women with breast cancer receiving chemotherapy in the experiment group with daily designed exercise programs had better quality of life scores compared with the control group in physical, psychological, and social dimension (30). Significant training effects have been observed in lower limb dynamic performance as well (31). The magnitude of incident loading during the observed training sessions seemed to be sufficiently high to increase bone mass in different subjects, suggesting that this kind of vigorous training regimen is feasible among breast cancer survivors, and could have the potential to prevent bone loss accompanying the adjuvant treatments of breast cancer (31).

Researchers have also reported that cancer survivors identified numerous improvements that they attributed to their participation in the exercise program (32). These included reduced fatigue and increased confidence, physical functioning, mental outlook, exercise participation and knowledge about exercise (32). Group theorists describe a "mutually shared field" that is generated when individuals who differ from one another, yet possess some commonality, are gathered (32). With a collective gathering and sharing of common ground, social interactions arise between individuals (or the group as a whole) that become motivational and inspirational. Through these social interactions, drawn from shared commonalities, change occurs.

While our findings do not provide specific exercise prescriptions for this group, they have shown that exercise had a positive effect on quality of life (33). These results are important to communicate to patients and their families, who may understandably be concerned that exercise will increase symptoms, including fatigue and discomfort. Analytical results of this study suggest several ways to increase exercise frequency in breast cancer survivors: encourage exercise as early as possible; improve health status and provide social support for exercise, especially in women older than 40 years, reduce exercise barriers and promote mental health, reinforce self-efficacy and positive expectations of exercise outcomes, and provide strategies for minimizing fatigue in early stages of rehabilitation (29). Researchers suggest that improving one's understanding of motivating factors would enable health professionals to develop effective exercise interventions in clinical settings (29). In addition to these recommendations, researchers have also investigated the effects of exercise in relation to the highest prevalence cancers such as lung, prostrate, and breast cancer.

Lung cancer and exercise

The past decade has seen a significant increase in research interest of the application of exercise following a cancer diagnosis (25). A study conducted investigated the efficacy of different types of exercise training on cardiorespiratory fitness in post-operative non-small cell lung cancer (NSCLC) patients. Approximately 26,000 individuals in the United States survive more than five years after the initial diagnosis of their operable disease (34). However, treatment-related morbidity is now recognized as a critical clinical issue in the management of NSCLC patients (34). The research indicates that a cardiorespiratory fitness may play a major role in ameliorating acute and insidious treatment-related toxicity. In NSCLC patients, aerobic training has been found to cause favorable adaptations in oxygen transport components. However, it is important to note that aerobic training used alone may be insufficient in reducing muscle atrophy and cachexia associated with conventional cancer treatments (34). According to Jones et al. (34) NSCLC patients have a significantly marked reduction in VO_{2peak}. Furthermore, pre-operative VO_{2peak} is now becoming a major area of research interest for its use in determining perioperative and postoperative complication risk. It was found that pre-operative VO_{2peak} is a strong independent clinical measurement that can be used to predict overall survival in NSCLC surgical patients (34). Pre-operative VO2 thus being such a powerful determinant of good prognosis, perhaps lifestyle changes throughout the course and after cancer treatment may extend the same prospective benefits to those who take initiative to improve physical fitness after diagnosis.

Observational studies suggest that regular exercise (i.e., 30 minutes of aerobic exercise at least five days/week) may be associated with significant reductions in cancer specific mortality among patients with early breast and colorectal cancer. A study conducted examined 25 patients with advanced lung cancer who underwent an exercise program, the authors found that exercise played a significant role in reducing lung cancer symptoms and improvement in the six-minute walk test (35). However, secondary to lung cancer, patients commonly experience symptoms such as dyspnea and severe coughing which diminishes exercise tolerance, which is an important consideration when helping lung cancer patients cope with dyspnea, and other disease related complications (2). Direction on different forms of activity that may be out of the classical schema of working out should be offered to these patients to build them up to a level of healthy tolerance for more demanding exercise.

Prostate cancer and exercise

Most prostate cancer patients are treated with androgen deprivation therapy (ADT), this serves to reduce the proliferation of prostate cells by lowering testosterone levels (36). However, ADT is often used in conjunction with radiation therapy and is associated with decrements in strength, aerobic capacity, decreased balance, gain in fat mass, elevated levels of fatigue, deterioration in bone health, and cognitive impairment (36). Exercise can be used as an effective resource to manage the adverse effects of ADT (36).

A study conducted examined the effects of resistance exercise for men on ADT, and it was reported that resistance exercise can prevent ADT induced increase in body fat and preserve whole-body lean mass (37). In a second study conducted by Segal et al. (37), the effects of resistance training combined with aerobic exercise were investigated in men with prostate cancer receiving radiation therapy coupled with or without ADT (37). During the intervention, the researchers found that upper and lower body strength were significantly improved in the resistance exercise group. Aerobic exercise can be used to prevent feelings of fatigue that are commonly associated with men undergoing ADT coupled with radiation therapy (37). It is important to note that a common trend observed in all the intervention studies for men on ADT is the lack of weight reduction, and lipolysis (37). Despite ADT's role in lowering testosterone, it is required to inhibit adipogenesis and stimulate lipolysis (38). Therefore, the increased caloric expenditure associated with exercise may not offset the regulatory effects of the hormonal imbalance. However, weight control can be managed using routine exercise, and a well-balanced diet (38).

Exercise and physical activity in breast cancer survivors

Regular exercise and physical activity in breast cancer survivors has been associated with decreased cancer-related fatigue, improvements in immune system function, increased quality of life, and an overall reduced incidence of cancer reoccurrence (39). Additionally, exercise intensity may play a vital role in breast cancer survival rates. Moderate-high intensity exercise has been found to decrease the risk of breast cancer related death (39). However, despite these findings only half of breast cancer survivors engage in regular exercise.

In a recent randomized controlled trial, it was found that weightlifting programs reduced the symptoms associated with severe lymphedema in breast cancer survivors (40). A progressive weightlifting program for breast cancer survivors was also found to increase muscular strength and reduce the severity of symptoms of aggressive lymphedema in the arms and hands (40). It is important to note that after undergoing breast cancer surgery fear has been identified as a major barrier to physical activity in women (40). Researchers reported that side effects of conventional cancer treatment for post-operative breast cancer survivors such as fatigue, neuropathy, anxiety, self-esteem, and fear of lymphedema contributed to barriers concerning physical activity (40). Therefore, the research suggests that health care providers need to be aware of factors that may serve as barriers to exercise in breast cancer survivors when developing a rehabilitation plan. Being that fear has been identified as a major barrier to physical activity in breast cancer survivors, the impact of exercise on anxiety states has gained much attention.

Breast cancer and exercise on anxiety state

In previous investigations, breast cancer survivors have reported higher states of anxiety coupled with a sense of no control in their world (40). This has been the driving force supporting the use of exercise as an alternative nonmedical option that can help reduce anxiety levels in breast cancer survivors (40). Breast cancer survivors have reported a reduction in anxiety when exercising (40). A study served to examine whether acute exercise reduces state anxiety in breast cancer survivors versus those without a cancer diagnosis, and it was reported that the main effects of exercise on anxiety levels in breast cancer survivors were significant (40). Therefore, it was concluded that exercise at moderate, and light intensities, may provide clinicians with another strategy in effectively reducing anxiety levels in breast cancer survivors. Further research is warranted concerning optimal testing, and prescriptions methods, for breast cancer survivors.

Conclusion

The research suggests that concerns about the side effects and interactions between complementary modalities, and conventional treatments, are rising (2). As a result of the insufficient scientific evidence, there remains a lack of dosage guidelines for high-dose antioxidant therapy. Furthermore, antioxidant therapy has raised concerns regarding its influence upon chemotherapy and radiation, which can depend on oxidative damage to tumor cells for the desired anticancer effects (2). Studies investigating complementary therapies such as tai chi, yoga, acupuncture, and meditation indicate they may enhance the effects of conventional medical treatment. Further studies are warranted to understand the underlying nature of how these therapies express their effects in cancer patient populations. Regarding physical activity, the research indicates that regular exercise has a positive effect on quality of life, cancer-related fatigue, mood, and emotional distress in cancer patients (26). Lifestyle interventions that promote improvements in diet and exercise behaviors have also been proposed to ameliorate the adverse effects of cancer and its treatment. Additional research is warranted concerning the interactions between the acute and long-term side effects of complementary therapies, conventional medical treatments, and physical activity for cancer survivors as cancer treatments continue to evolve.

References

[1] Young-McCaughan S, Mays MZ, Arzola SM, Yoder LH, Dramiga SA, Leclerc KM. Change in exercise tolerance, activity and sleep patterns, and quality of life in patients with cancer participating in a structured exercise program including commentary by Mock V. Oncol Nurs Forum 2003;30(3):441454.

[2] Anderson JG, Taylor AG. Use of complementary therapies for cancer symptom management: Results of the 2007 National Health Interview Survey. J Altern Complement Med 2012;18(3):235-41.

[3] Eisenberg DM, Davis RB, Ettner SL,Appel S, Wilkey S, Rompay M, Kessler RC. Trends in alternative medicine use in the United States, 1990-1997: Results from a follow up national survey. JAMA 1998;280:1569-75.

[4] Pierce JP, Stefanick ML, Flatt SW, Natarjan L, Sternfeld B, Madlensky L, et al. Greater survival after breast cancer in physically active women with high vegetable-fruit intake regardless of obesity. J Clin Oncol 2007;25(17):2345-51.

[5] Hilakivi-Clarke L, Andrade JE, Helferich, W. Is soy consumption good or bad for the breast? J Nutrition 2010;140(12):2326-34S.

[6] Guha N, Kwan ML, Queensberry CP, Weltzien EK, Castillo AL, Caan BJ. Soy isoflavones and risk of cancer recurrence in a cohort of breast cancer survivors: The Life After Cancer Epidemiology study. Breast Cancer Res Treat 2009;118(2):395-405.

[7] Suhail N, Bilal N, Khan HY, Hasan S, Sharma S, Khan F, Mansoor T, Banu N. Effect of vitamins C and E on antioxidant status of breast-cancer patients undergoing chemotherapy. J Clin Pharm Ther 2012;37(1):22-6.

[8] Ross L, Fletcher A, Anderson MC, Meade SA, Powe B, Howard D. Complementary and Alternative Medicine (CAM) Use among with a history of prostate cancer. J Cultural Divers 2012;19(4):143-50.

[9] Drisko JA, Chapman J, Hunter VJ. The use of antioxidants with first-line chemotherapy in two cases of ovarian cancer. J Am Coll Nutr 2003;22:118-23.

[10] Galantino ML, Callens ML,Cardena GJ, Piela NL,James J. Tai chi for well-being of breast cancer survivors with aromatase inhibitor-associated arthralgias: A feasibility study. Altern Ther Health Med 2013;19(6):38-44.

[11] Burstein HJ, Winer EP. Aromatase inhibitors and arthralgias: A new frontier in symptom management for breast cancer survivors. J Clin Oncol 2007;25(25):3797-9.

[12] Peppone LJ, Mustian KM, Janelsins MC, Palesh OG, Rosier RN, Piazza KM, Purnell JQ,Darling TV, Morrow, GR. Effects of a structured weight-bearing exercise program on bone metabolism among breast cancer survivors: a feasibility trial. J Clin Breast Cancer 2010;10(3):224-9.

[13] Sprod LK, Janelsins MC, Palesh, OG, Carrol JK, Heckler CE, Peppone LJ, Mohile SG, Morrow GR, Mustain KM. Health related quality of life and biomarkers in breast cancer survivors participating in Tai chi chuan. J Cancer Survivors 2012;6(2):146-54.

[14] Reid-Arndt SA, Matsuda S, Cox CR. Tai chi effects on neuropsychological, emotional, and physical functioning following cancer treatment: A pilot study. Complement Ther Clin Pract 2012;18(1):26-30.

[15] Smith BW, Shelley BM, Dalen J, Wiggins K, Toolet E, Bernard J. A pilot study comparing the effects of mindfulness-based and cognitive behavioral stress reduction. J Altern Complement Med 2008;14(3):251-8.

[16] Dhruva A, Miashowski C, Abrams D, Acree M, Cooper B, Goodman S, Hecht F. Yoga breathing for cancer chemotherapy-associated symptoms and quality of life: results of a pilot randomized controlled trial. J Altern Complement Med 2011;18(5):473-9.

[17] Upadhyay DK, Malhotra V, Sarkar D, Prajapati R. Effect of alternate nostril breathing exercise on cardiorespiratory functions. Nepal Med Coll J 2008;10(1):25-7.

[18] Maguire GP, Lee EG, Bevington DJ, Kuchermann CS, Crabtree RJ, Cornell CE. Psychiatric problems in the first year after mastectomy. BMJ 1978;1 (6118): 9630965.

[19] Zhang J, Yang K, Tian J, Wang C. Effects of yoga on psychologic function and quality of life in women with breast cancer: A meta-analysis of randomized controlled trials. J Altern Complement Med 2012;18(11):994-002.

[20] Jaung-Geng L, Yi-Hung C. The role of acupuncture in cancer supportive care. Am J Chinese Med 2012;40(2):219-29.

[21] Filshie J. The non-drug treatment of neuralgic and neuropathic pain of malignancy. Cancer Survivors 1988;7(1):161-93.

[22] Braga FP, Lemos Junior CA., Alves, FA, Migliari DA. Acupuncture for the prevention of radiation-induced xerostomia in patients with head and neck cancer. Brazilian Oral Res 2011;25(2):180-5.

[23] Chambers SK, Smith DP, Berry M, Lepore SJ, Foley E, Clutton S, McDowall R, Occhipinti S, Frydenberg M, Gardiner RA. A randomized controlled trial of a mindfulness intervention for men with advanced prostate cancer. BMC Cancer 2013;13:89.

[24] Speca M, Carlson LE, Goodey E, Angen M. A randomized, wait-list controlled clinical trial: the effect of a mindfulness meditation-based stress reduction program on mood and symptoms of stress in cancer outpatients. Psychosomat Med 2000;62(5):613-22.

[25] Pekmezi DW, Demark WW. Updated evidence in support of diet and exercise interventions in cancer survivors. Acta Oncologica 2011;50:167–78.

[26] O'Mathúna DP. Exercise during and after cancer treatment. Chinese J Integr Med 2012; 15(7):73-80.

[27] Litterini AJ, Jette DU. Exercise for managing cancer-related fatigue. J Phys Ther 2010; 91(3):301-4.

[28] Wu H, Dodd, M J, Cho MH. Patterns of fatigue and effect of exercise in patients receiving chemotherapy for breast cancer. Oncol Nurs Forum 2008; 35(5):90-9.

[29] Hsu HT, Dodd MJ, Guo SE, Lee KA, Hwang SL, Lai YH. Predictors of exercise frequency in breast cancer survivors in Taiwan. J Clin Nurs 2011;20(13-14):1923-35.

[30] Maryam A, Fazlollah A, Eesa M, Ebrahim H, Abbas VF. The effect of designed exercise programme on quality of life in women with breast cancer receiving chemotherapy. Scand J Caring Sci 2010;24(2):251-8.
[31] Nikander R, Sievänen H, Ojala K, Oivanen T, Kellokumpu-Lehtinen PL, Saarto T. Effect of a vigorous aerobic regimen on physical performance in breast cancer patients—a randomized controlled pilot trial. Acta Oncol 2007;46(2):181-6.
[32] Spence RR, Heesch KC, Brown WJ. Colorectal cancer survivors' exercise experiences and preferences: qualitative findings from an exercise rehabilitation programme immediately after chemotherapy. Eur J Cancer Care 2011;20(2):257-66.
[33] Sander AP, Wilson J, Izzo N, Mountford SA, Hayes KW. Factors that affect decisions about physical activity and exercise in survivors of breast cancer: a qualitative study. Phys Ther 2012;92(4):525-36.
[34] Jones LW, Eves ND, Kraus WE, Potti A, Crawford J, Blumenthal JA, Peterson BL, Douglas PS. The lung cancer exercise training study: a randomized trial of aerobic training, resistance training, or both in postsurgical lung cancer patients: Rationale and design. BMC Cancer 2010;10):155.
[35] Temel JS, Greer JA, Goldberg S, Vogel PD, Sullivan M, Pirl WF, Lynch TJ, Christiani DC, Smith MR. A structured exercise program for patients with advanced non-small cell lung cancer. J Thoracic Oncol 2009;4(5):595-601.
[36] Shahinian VB, Kuo YF, Freeman JL, Goodwin JS. Risk of the "androgen deprivation syndrome" in men receiving androgen deprivation for prostate cancer. Arch Intern Med 2006;166(4):465-71.
[37] Segal RJ, Reid RD, Courneya KS, Sigal RJ, Kenny GP, Prud'Homme DG, Malone SC, Wells GA, Scott CG, Slovinec D'Angelo ME. Randomized controlled trial of resistance or aerobic exercise in men receiving radiation therapy for prostate cancer. J Clin Oncol 2009;27(3):344-51.
[38] De Pergola G. The adipose tissue metabolism: role of testosterone and dehydroepiandrosterone. Int J Obes Relat Metabol Disord 2000;24:59-63.
[39] Friedenreich CM, Gregory J, Kopciuk KA, Mackey JR, Courneya KS. Prospective cohort study of lifetime physical activity and breast cancer survival. Int J Cancer 2009;124(8):1954-62.
[40] Schmitz KH, Ahmed RL, Troxel A, Cheville A, Smith R, Lewis-Grant L, Bryan CJ, Williams-Smith CT, Greene QP. Weight lifting in women with breast-cancer–related lymphedema. New Engl J Med 2009;361(7):664-73.

Chapter 7

Sudden cardiac death in basketball players in the United States: Public health implications

Travis Pearson[1], MD, MPH
Victoriann Jones[1], BS
Evan DeMonte[1], BM, NRP
Chanpreet Mangat[1], BSc
Jounaidou Mbouemboue[1], BSc, MSc
Osazee Eguagie[2], MD, PGCME
and Emmanuel O Keku[1], MD, MA, MSPH
[1]Department of Public Health and Preventive Medicine, St George's University, School of Medicine, St George, Grenada, West Indies
[2]Department of Pathophysiology, St George's University, School of Medicine, St George, Grenada, West Indies

Abstract

This literature review examined the different etiologies leading to sudden cardiac death in basketball players and the interventions that different institutions have taken to reduce its incidence. Methods: The review was conducted using search engines including, but not limited to, Google Scholar, Medline, EBSCO Host, and PubMed. The keywords used to find potentially relevant articles included "sudden death," "sudden cardiac death," "sudden cardiac arrest," and "basketball." Results: Literature suggests that sudden cardiac death can be caused by an enormous release of catecholamines during the physiological stress response which activates adrenergic receptors. This could lead to ventricular arrhythmias, myocardial ischemia due to coronary vasospasm, and coronary artery

In: Public Health
Editors: Emmanuel O Keku and Joav Merrick
ISBN: 979-8-89113-083-8

occlusion leading to myocardial infarction. The most frequent etiology leading to sudden cardiac arrest and death is hypertrophic cardiomyopathy. The current protocol for screening recommended by the American Heart Association consists of a personal and family history along with a physical examination. While the protocol for screening varies among high schools and colleges, the National Basketball Association has a standardized protocol for all 30 teams involving: history, physical examination, blood work, electrocardiogram, and echocardiogram testing. Conclusion: This literature review suggests that the current protocol for cardiac screening at the high school and college levels is insufficient and should incorporate more testing, including electrocardiogram.

Keywords: sudden death, sudden cardiac death, sudden cardiac arrest, basketball, United States

Introduction

When talking about "sudden death" in sports, the first thing that comes to mind is whichever team scores the next point or goal wins the game. However, the medical significance of this expression is much grimmer than the simple outcome of a game.

Sudden cardiac death (SCD), or sudden cardiac arrest (SCA), is defined as "the sudden, unexpected loss of heart function, breathing, and consciousness" (1). It may arise from several underlying heart conditions, and as the name implies - can occur in an instant and without warning.

SCD is one of the many cardiovascular diseases that have been the leading cause of death around the world. Alone, sudden cardiac death claims about 350,000 lives per year in the United States. Studies show that 80% of sudden cardiac arrest cases occur outside of the hospital and out of those, less than 30% are attended to by either medical personnel or bystanders. Nine out of ten Americans who experienced a sudden cardiac arrest have died. SCD can happen to anyone regardless of their health and level of fitness. This applies especially to young athletes, who are 2.5 times more susceptible to the occurrence of SCD than nonathletes (1). This higher prevalence in athletes can be explained by the considerable amounts of stress athletes place on their heart during intense sports, such as basketball, soccer, or football (2). Due to a tremendously low survival rate, the difficulty in its diagnosis, and the relative lack of access to immediate medical care upon occurrence, SCD is considered a serious public health issue, even more so when it affects young people.

One case that gained national attention is the death of Hank Gathers, a 23-year-old black male collegiate basketball player at Loyola Marymount University in Los Angeles, California. As a junior, he led the nation in scoring and rebounding in 1989 and was hailed as one of the top NBA prospects going into his senior season. In March 1990 during a conference tournament game, Gathers collapsed after scoring a dunk and stopped breathing. Soon after, he was pronounced dead. He had a similar syncopal episode earlier in the season in December 1989 when he collapsed during the game after sprinting the entire length of the court. After running extensive cardiological diagnostics, he was found to have exercise-induced ventricular tachyarrhythmia, worsened by the extremely high tempo "run and gun" offense that his team plays, and was prescribed propranolol, a beta blocker (3). After a few weeks, Gathers was allowed to return to competitive basketball so long as he adhered to the medication regimen (3).

Because of the nature of SCD, it is often difficult to predict what exactly causes it. An analysis of 1866 cases in the US between 1980 and 2006 showed that 1049, or 56% of them could be caused by cardiovascular diseases. Of those 1049, 690 could be linked to 44 cardiovascular diseases with reliability (4). A common limitation among studies concerning SCD seems to be the inability to identify a definitive cause of death in certain cases (5). Maron et al. (4) found in their study that in many cases, the cause of death related to SCD could not be reliably determined by preparticipation screening, even with ECG. Young athletes who die because of sudden cardiac arrest have usually not been diagnosed with any heart disorders prior to death, which also lends to the unpredictability of the disease. In the study by Maron et al. (4) only 75 of the 1866 cases had an earlier diagnosis of a cardiac disorder.

The sport being played at the time of death as well as the level of participation can also be factors for SCD. High intensity sports are seen to contribute the most to SCDs. The sports contributing the most to SCD in the U.S. are basketball and football (4, 5). However, those results may be biased due to the popularity of those sports in the US as soccer, the most popular sport in Europe and most of the world, is seen to be the greatest contributor to SCD in those countries (6). SCDs seem to occur most often at the high school level, followed by middle school and collegiate levels (4, 6). About 1 in 44,000 athletes taking part in collegiate sports in the U.S. dies from sudden cardiac arrest each year (5). Among US collegiate athletes, increased risk of SCD is seen among males, African Americans, and basketball players. Risk among male basketball players has been seen to be about 10 times greater than the overall athlete population (7). The sport of basketball will be the particular focus of this research, with the goal being to raise awareness and help reduce the incidence of SCD through identifying the etiologies and pathophysiology of SCD and providing recommendations to eventually reach this goal.

Methods

Studies, articles, and presentations that touch upon the subject of sudden cardiac death in basketball players were collectively analyzed. Numerous search engines were used for this paper, including but not limited to, Google Scholar, Medline, EBSCO Host, and PubMed. The keywords used to find relevant articles included "sudden death," "sudden cardiac death," "sudden cardiac arrest," and "basketball." Further analysis was performed, reviewing each article to determine and improve relevance with the understanding that most articles would be about athletes in general and not limited to basketball players. Searches were focused on material from the past 15 years, however some articles from as far back as 1993 were considered too relevant to the subject matter to exclude.

Results

There are several etiologies that can predispose an individual to SCD which incorporate a common mechanism. This mechanism involves the activation of the sympathetic nervous system and the resulting large release of catecholamines during the physiological stress response. The release of catecholamines leads to the activation of α- and β-adrenoreceptors, with the action of the latter being critical to the possible development of SCD. The activation of the β-adrenoceptors leads to a significant increase of calcium influx into the myocardial cells during the cardiac action potential as well as further release of calcium from the sarcoplasmic reticulum. The change in how the calcium is managed can eventually induce ventricular arrhythmias commonly associated with SCD. The activation of α-adrenoreceptors through increased levels of catecholamines can result in coronary spasm causing myocardial ischemia, which can also contribute to etiologies involved in SCD. The catecholamines themselves can also be subject to auto-oxidation, which can damage the cardiomyocytes. They are also shown to increase platelet aggregation & atherosclerotic plaque formation, which can increase the risk of coronary artery occlusion and result in a myocardial infarction (8).

Hypertrophic cardiomyopathy

The most frequent cause of sudden cardiac death is hypertrophic cardiomyopathy (HCM), which is a condition that affects one in every five hundred people in the general population (1:500). This data is based on echocardiographic population studies in which a sizable portion of the affected subjects has not been clinically diagnosed (9). HCM can be difficult to accurately diagnose as it occurs in patients of all ages and most patients remain clinically stable or asymptomatic (10). Diagnosis of HCM requires echocardiographic evidence of a hypertrophied, non-dilated left ventricle in the absence of another cardiac or systemic disease that could produce a similar degree of hypertrophy. Hypertrophy of the left ventricle is defined as a wall thickness of equal to or greater than fifteen millimeters (≥15mm) in adult index patients or the equivalent wall thickness relative to body-surface area in children (11, 12). The magnitude of left ventricular hypertrophy has been shown to be a strong and independent predictor of the risk of SCD in patients with HCM (12). Other risk factors of HCM may include a family history of SCD, syncope, non-sustained ventricular tachycardia, and abnormal blood pressure in response to exercise (13). It is most often a genetic disorder, inherited primarily as an autosomal dominant trait, meaning an individual would need only one copy of the mutant gene to become affected. Over 400 mutations of at least 24 genes associated with HCM have been discovered as recently as 2010 (11).

Coronary artery anomalies

After HCM, coronary artery anomalies are the next most common cause of SCD, and they are prevalent in about 2.5% of the population (4, 14, 15). Coronary artery anomalies may occur as part of a complex congenital malformation, or it may occur as an isolated abnormality. One type of anomaly occurs when a coronary artery arises from the wrong aortic sinus; the most common occurrence being the left main coronary artery originating from the right sinus of Valsalva (14). SCD due to coronary artery anomalies is thought to be related to myocardial ischemia, and the course of the artery is theorized to be of pathological significance. The first segment of an anomalous coronary artery can travel between the aorta and the pulmonary trunk, which can cause compression and squeezing of the artery during physical activity and lead to myocardial ischemia (16). Another theorized pathological mechanism is the acute takeoff of the artery from the sinus, resulting in a slit-like orifice at the point of origin, which differs from the normal circular-like orifice and can lead to kinking and decreased blood flow during exercise (16, 17). Although individuals with coronary artery anomalies can be asymptomatic until exertion, the most common symptoms associated with these defects include syncope, angina and palpitations (16, 18). As with HCM, coronary artery anomalies are not usually identified unless suspicion is extremely high (18). Certain variants of coronary artery anomalies may be associated with a greater risk of SCD as suggested in some studies, but further investigation may be necessary for validity (16, 18).

Myocarditis

Myocarditis accounts for 5-22% of SCD cases in athletes under 35 years of age (19). In more than 50% of all cases, Coxsackie B virus is the cause of myocarditis (17). Affected individuals may present with dyspnea, orthopnea, cough, and exercise intolerance. The infected myocardium can become inflamed, which can potentially cause a terminal arrhythmia or can lead to a heart block through involvement of the conduction system (17).

Other causes

Fatal cardiac arrhythmias can occur due to irregularities in the conduction system. The most common abnormalities involving the conduction system that are associated with SCD are Wolff-Parkinson-White syndrome (WPW), long QT syndrome (LQTS), and Brugada syndrome (BrS). Other causes involve hereditary connective tissue diseases, the most common one being Marfan syndrome. Marfan syndrome is an autosomal dominant disorder occurring in about 1 in 10,000 people. Defective elastic fibers within the connective tissue can lead to progressive dilatation of the aortic root, dislocation of the eye lens, and hyperextensible joints in addition to the classical findings of long, thin limbs and tall stature. Aortic root dilatation puts affected individuals at a greater risk of SCD and can lead to a complete dissection or rupture of the aorta along with subsequent mediastinal hemorrhage, pericardial tamponade, coronary artery dissection, or acute aortic insufficiency with congestive heart failure (17).

Commotio cordis

Blunt, nonpenetrating, and unintentional trauma to the chest can trigger ventricular fibrillation, leading to SCD. This occurrence is known as commotio cordis, or "concussion of the heart." Ventricular fibrillation occurs because the trauma alters the electrical stability of the myocardium. Studies show the blow must occur during the ventricular repolarization phase of the cardiac cycle (20).

How race affects diagnosis

As difficult as diagnosis for factors leading to SCD can be, there seems to be a disparity in identification between whites and African Americans. According to a study, HCM among African Americans was seven times more likely to be identified at autopsy compared to identification during life. The disparity is likely due to disproportionate access to cardiovascular medical care, in large part because of socioeconomic factors, and misdiagnosis of HCM-related left ventricular hypertrophy as attributed to systemic hypertension (21).

Protocols

It is undoubtedly difficult to predict any occurrence of SCD. Most predisposing etiologies are troublesome to correctly diagnose, which further adds to the unpredictability of SCD. It remains important to identify and diagnose any high-risk individuals playing basketball and develop the proper approach so that the risk of SCD is significantly reduced.

Though there is universal agreement that screening, especially pre-participation screening, should be utilized to help detect any cardiovascular diseases, there seems to be debate as to what the approach to screening should be. The current protocol in the US as recommended by the American Heart Association (AHA) consists of a 12-point history and physical exam. The 12-

point history includes five elements of personal history, three elements of family history, and four elements of the physical exam. The limitation in this protocol is that the history and physical exam would not be sufficient to effectively identify at-risk individuals since many present as asymptomatic (22). The European Society of Cardiology (ESC), on the other hand, does include 12-lead electrocardiography in addition to a detailed medical history and physical exam in their protocol (23). In 2006, the National Basketball Association (NBA) installed a protocol requiring standardized cardiac screening for every player, becoming the first major professional sports league in the US to do so. The installation was spurred into action due to the death of Jason Collier, a 28-year-old center who was playing for the Atlanta Hawks. The NBA's screening process includes detailed personal and family medical histories, a physical exam, blood work, and three heart tests: an ECG, a resting echocardiogram, and a stress echocardiogram. These tests are administered annually and must be completed for a player to participate in training camp. Before the standardized protocol, all 30 NBA teams were allowed to set their own parameters for cardiac screening (24).

The National Collegiate Athletic Association (NCAA) assembled a task force in September 2014 to decide how to best handle pre-participation screening and create guidelines for how to deal with a SCA in progress. Though they have not recommended screening with an ECG to be implemented across all institutions, they did provide best practices to institutions that choose to require the tests. The consensus among the task force was that a well-rehearsed and effective emergency plan should be in place to reduce the risk of death, which includes available and working automatic external defibrillators (AEDs) during practice and play (25). In 2015, Brain Hainline, the first-ever chief medical officer of the NCAA announced a plan that would have required all student athletes to receive ECGs but eventually withdrew that plan when he received backlash from team physicians from over 100 institutions (26).

At the high school level, athletes must undergo a preparticipation physical evaluation (PPE) every 1-3 years or depending on state requirements. The PPE follows the standards of the AHA, consisting of, at the minimum, a history, and a physical exam. (27) The lack of standardization at the college and high school levels is another shortcoming. For example, 35% of states allow examiners that do not have the proper cardiovascular evaluation training to conduct the PPE (28).

Discussion

Cardiovascular screening of all basketball players (from high school to professional level) should occur prior to participation as a critical step in diagnosis and prevention. This pre-participation screening should include extensive cardiovascular history with a physical exam, along with the use of diagnostic tools such as an electrocardiogram (ECG) and an echocardiogram. ECG screening has been proven to have increased sensitivity in detecting cardiovascular diseases and is also a cost-effective measure. Studies showed that adding the ECG to the previously recommended practice of taking history and completing a physical showed to be $42,900 (~2.06 life years per 1,000 athletes) per life year saved, which is acceptable by US standards (29, 28). Screening with diagnostic tools such as an ECG should be performed by an accredited physician specializing in cardiology or sport medicine (23). Management of positive findings during screenings should be handled on a person-to-person basis. Treatment options should include lifestyle modifications, antiarrhythmic drugs such as amiodarone, beta-blockers, restriction of competitive activity, and implantable cardioverter-defibrillator therapy (30). Athletes should be made aware of the risks and benefits with each treatment option, as well as the perceived risk of continued participation in basketball. Physicians should also closely follow-up with these athletes and manage their treatment according to the situation (30).

For example, a nationwide systematic preparticipation screening program was implemented in Italy in 1982 for all competitive athletes, which included family and personal history, physical examination, and a 12-lead ECG with additional testing requested for athletes having positive findings. The program managed to reduce the incidence rate of SCD among young competitive athletes in the Veneto region of Italy by 89% (31). The limitation in the European Society of Cardiology's model, however, is that though it is commonly accepted worldwide, it is not standardized. It is also considered to be overly expensive and impractical to perform on a routine basis, despite its apparent cost-effectiveness (23).

Despite the cost-effectiveness of using an ECG in addition to a detailed medical history and physical exam, it is still possible to miss an etiology that can predispose an athlete to sudden cardiac death and should not be the sole method used to curtail the incidence of SCD, there must also be protocol in place to identify and respond to cardiac incidences quickly and adequately. A case of SCD can happen at any moment, preparation for the worst possible outcome should be the onus. Cardiopulmonary resuscitation (CPR) and the use of an AED is a skill possessed by most if not all emergency responders, however, CPR and AED training should not be limited to team physicians and emergency responders but should be extended to trainers and coaches and even the players themselves (25). Capucci et al. (32) suggested that use of an AED alone, without CPR, can triple the survival rate of SCA outside of the hospital because it reduces the response and intervention time, is cost-effective, and removes any concerns bystanders might have about giving mouth-to-mouth contact. The time between the athletes' collapse and defibrillation is considered the single greatest determinant of survival after SCA. With every minute that passes without defibrillation, the survival rate decreases up to 10% (33). AED programs at high schools have been proven to provide a high survival rate for both student athletes and adults who suffer SCA on the school grounds (33, 34). Though many states have legislation that mandates every school has at least one working AED on site, this should be implemented across all states across America along with the proper training of students, teachers, and athletic directors. As related to basketball and other sports, an AED should be readily available on the sideline of each practice and game. Basic Life Support (BLS) courses should be a part of the curriculum for all student-athletes attending high schools, colleges, and universities. If there were more personnel trained in CPR and AED use, individuals would be more prepared in dealing with SCA and prevention of SCD.

Conclusion

Though SCD has low incidence in the U.S., it is still a major public health problem, especially among young basketball players and athletes in general. Identifying the causes and risk factors and knowing what to do in that situation can potentially decrease the chance that an SCA could occur. Through the combination of primary (AED and CPR) and secondary (pre-participation screening) prevention, basketball players should have less to worry about when playing the sport they love.

Conflict of interest

The author reports no conflicts of interest.

References

[1] Higgins J, Andino A. Soccer and sudden cardiac death in young competitive athletes: A review. J Sports Med 2013;2013(7):1-7.

[2] Link M, Estes N. Sudden cardiac death in the athlete: Bridging the gaps between evidence, policy, and practice. Circulation 2012;125(20):2511-6.

[3] Maron B. Sudden death in young athletes - Lessons from the Hank Gathers affair. New Engl J Med 1993;329(1):55-7.

[4] Maron B, Doerer J, Haas T, Tierney D, Mueller F. Sudden deaths in young competitive athletes: Analysis of 1866 deaths in the United States, 1980-2006. Circulation 2009;119(8):1085-92.

[5] Harmon K, Asif I, Klossner D, Drezner J. Incidence of sudden cardiac death in National Collegiate Athletic Association athletes. Circulation 2011;123(15):1594-600.

[6] Chandra N, Bastiaenen R, Papadakis M, Sharma S. Sudden cardiac death in young athletes. JACC 2013;61(10):1027-40.

[7] Wasfy M, Hutter A, Weiner R. Sudden cardiac death in athletes. Methodist Debakey Cardiovasc J 2016;12(2):76-80.

[8] Goyal V, Jassal D, Dhalla N. Pathophysiology and prevention of sudden cardiac death. Can J Physiol Pharmacol 2015;94(3):237-44.

[9] Semsarian C, Ingles J, Maron M, Maron B. New perspectives on the prevalence of hypertrophic cardiomyopathy. JACC 2015;65(12):1249-54.

[10] Stroumpoulis K, Pantazopoulos I, Xanthos T. Hypertrophic cardiomyopathy and sudden cardiac death. World J Cardiol 2010;2(9) 289-98.

[11] Lynge T, Risgaard B, Jabbari R, Glinge C, Bundgaard H, Maron B. et al. Cardiac symptoms before sudden cardiac death caused by hypertrophic cardiomyopathy: a nationwide study among the young in Denmark. Europace 2016;18(12):1801-8.

[12] Spirito P, Bellone P, Harris K, Bernabò P, Bruzzi P, Maron B. Magnitude of left ventricular hypertrophy and risk of sudden death in hypertrophic cardiomyopathy. New Engl J Med 2000; 342(24):1778-85.

[13] Dimitrow P, Chojnowska L, Rudzinski T, Piotrowski W, Ziolkowska L, Wojtarowicz A. et al. (2010). Sudden death in hypertrophic cardiomyopathy: old risk factors re-assessed in a new model of maximalized follow-up. Eur Heart J 2010;31(24):3084-93.

[14] Maron B. Sudden death in young athletes. New Engl J Med 2003;349(11):1064-75.

[15] McLarry J, Ferencik M, Shapiro M. Coronary artery anomalies: A pictorial review. Curr Cardiovasc Imaging Rep 2015 May 15;8:23.

[16] Frescura C, Basso C, Thiene G, Corrado D, Pennelli T, Angelini A, Daliento L. Anomalous origin of coronary arteries and risk of sudden death: A study based on an autopsy population of congenital heart disease. Hum Pathol 1998;29(7):689-95.

[17] Koester MC. A Review of sudden cardiac death in young athletes and strategies for preparticipation cardiovascular screening. J Athl Train 2001;36(2):197–204.

[18] Basso C, Maron B, Corrado D, Thiene G. Clinical profile of congenital coronary artery anomalies with origin from the wrong aortic sinus leading to sudden death in young competitive athletes. JACC 2000;35(6):1493-501.

[19] Frick M, Pachinger O, Pölzl G. Myokarditis als Ursache des plötzlichen Herztodes bei Sportlern. Herz 2009;34(4):299-304. [German]

[20] Maron B, Estes N. Commotio cordis. New Engl J Med 2010;362(10):917-27.

[21] Maron B, Carney K, Lever H, Lewis J, Barac I, Casey S, et al. Relationship of race to sudden cardiac death in competitive athletes with hypertrophic cardiomyopathy. JACC 2003;41(6):974-80.

[22] Asif I, Rao A, Drezner J. Sudden cardiac death in young athletes: what is the role of screening? Curr Opin Cardiol 2013;28(1):55-62.

[23] Sharif S, Elzaydi N, Hydock D. Analysis of pre-participation screening protocols for football players in Europe, USA, and Libya: possible implications for preventing sudden cardiac death. Turkish J Sports Med 2017;52(2):63-9.

[24] Beck, H. The N.B.A. Is the first league to begin standardized cardiac screening. New York Times 2006 Sep 17.

[25] Hainline B, Drezner J, Baggish A, Harmon K, Emery M, Myerburg R. et al. Interassociation consensus statement on cardiovascular care of college student-athletes. JACC 2016;67(25):2981-95.

[26] Terlep S. NCAA doctor backs off recommending heart tests for athletes. Wall Street Journal 2015 Apr 17.

[27] Toresdahl B, Rao A, Harmon K, Drezner J. Incidence of sudden cardiac arrest in high school student athletes on school campus. Heart Rhythm 2014;11(7):1190-4.

[28] Schmehil C, Malhotra D, Patel D. Cardiac screening to prevent sudden death in young athletes. Transl Pediatr 2017;6(3):199-206.

[29] Wheeler MT, Heidenreich PA, Froelicher VF, Hlatky MA, Ashley EA. Cost effectiveness of pre-participation screening for prevention of sudden cardiac death in young athletes. Ann Intern Med 2010;152(5):276–86.

[30] Corrado D, Basso C, Schiavon M, Pelliccia A, Thiene G. Pre-participation screening of young competitive athletes for prevention of sudden cardiac death. JACC 2008;52(24):1981-9.

[31] Corrado D, Basso C, Pavei A, Michieli P, Schiavon M, Thiene G. Trends in sudden cardiovascular death in young competitive athletes after implementation of a preparticipation screening program. JAMA 2006;296(13):1593.

[32] Capucci A, Aschieri D, Piepoli M, Bardy G, Iconomu E, Arvedi M. Tripling survival from sudden cardiac arrest via early defibrillation without traditional education in cardiopulmonary resuscitation. Circulation 2002;106(9):1065-70.

[33] Drezner J, Rao A, Heistand J, Bloomingdale M, Harmon K. Effectiveness of emergency response planning for sudden cardiac arrest in United States high schools with automated external defibrillators. Circulation 2009;120(6):518-25.

[34] Drezner J, Toresdahl B, Rao A, Huszti E, Harmon K. Outcomes from sudden cardiac arrest in US high schools: a 2-year prospective study from the National Registry for AED use in sports. Br J Sports Med 2013;47(18):1179-83.

Chapter 8

An evaluation of the effectiveness of ivermectin in chemoprophylaxis and the treatment of COVID-19 patients: A narrative review

Alvin Chitterman, MD, MPH
Deepak Kumar Palanichami, BSc
Anthony La, BA
Victor Adedara, BSc, MS
Lauren Orlando, MSc, PhD
Emmanuel O Keku, MD, MA, MSPH
and Abidemi Fasanmi*, MD, MPH, PhD
School of Medicine, Department of Public Health and Preventive Medicine, St George's University, St George, Grenada, West Indies

Abstract

Many drug trials have failed to produce reliable proof of efficacy in reducing the mortality and transmission of the COVID-19 virus. Apart from corticosteroids, there has been limited evidence on interventions that can prevent transmission and treat COVID-19 patients. Ivermectin has antiviral properties and is a safe, orally taken, and affordable drug. Therefore, evaluating ivermectin in chemoprophylaxis and treatment of COVID-19 patients would be necessary. This was a narrative review paper to evaluate the effectiveness of ivermectin in chemoprophylaxis

* Corresponding Author's Email: afasanmi@sgu.edu; Abidemi Fasanmi, MD, MPH, PhD., Assistant Professor, School of Medicine, Department of Public Health, and Preventive Medicine, POBox 7, St. George, Grenada, West Indies.

In: Public Health
Editors: Emmanuel O Keku and Joav Merrick
ISBN: 979-8-89113-083-8

and the treatment of COVID-19 patients. Using the Google Scholar database, Medline Plus, and ScienceDirect, a literature search was conducted with the keywords "COVID-19 treatment and prophylaxis" and "ivermectin treatment and prophylaxis for COVID-19 disease." Regular ivermectin use in two randomized controlled trials (RCTs) and five observational studies has shown a statistically significantly reduced risk of COVID-19 transmission in prophylaxis trials, $P < 0.05$. Ten RCTs have shown a statistically significant reduction in time to patient recovery, time for viral clearance, and reduced mortality, $P < 0.05$. The efficacy of two RCTs showed insignificant results $P > 0.05$. Ivermectin is beneficial in treating and reducing COVID-19 transmissions. However, a meta-analysis is recommended to determine the pooled effect of ivermectin efficacy on COVID-19 patients.

Keywords: Coronavirus, COVID-19, SARS – CoV2, ivermectin

Introduction

Ivermectin, discovered from the streptomyces bacterium in the 1970s in Japan, has been used extensively worldwide (1). It was first introduced as an antiparasitic drug, effective against parasites, including gastrointestinal roundworms, lungworms, mites, lice and horn flies (2). Ivermectin is a Food and Drug Administration-approved antiparasitic drug in animals (3). Despite being introduced as a veterinary drug, ivermectin has been used since 1988 to treat onchocerciasis (River blindness), a severely debilitating vector-borne parasitic disease which has been targeted for elimination worldwide. The successful use of Ivermectin in addressing this disease has improved the health, nutrition, and well-being of the affected populations (4).

Ivermectin is notably well known for two global elimination campaigns. It has almost eliminated onchocerciasis and lymphatic filariasis, two diseases that significantly affected the health of billions of disadvantaged populations (5). This is the reason ivermectin discoverers were awarded the Nobel Prize in medicine in 2015 (6).

Ivermectin also has antiviral and anti-inflammatory properties (7, 8). Ivermectin has shown efficacy against several RNA viruses, including human immunodeficiency virus (HIV-1), dengue virus, and SARS-CoV2 (9). It inhibited SARS-CoV2 in vitro with almost undetectable viral material after 48 hours (10). In further molecular studies, ivermectin was shown to competitively bind to the host receptors' binding region on SARS-CoV2 (11).

High ivermectin binding activity to spike protein S1 region domain on SARS-CoV2 can limit the binding of the SARS-CoV2 to ACE 2 host receptors decreasing the virus's entry into host cells (12). Gudadappanavar and Benni (13) have shown that ivermectin inhibits viral replication by targeting the SARS-CoV2 RNA-dependent RNA polymerase.

Apart from corticosteroids, there has been limited evidence on interventions that can prevent transmission and treat COVID-19 patients. Considering the existing potential mechanisms of actions of ivermectin against SARS-CoV2, it is essential to review the literature for evidence of the effectiveness of Ivermectin in the prophylaxis and treatment against SARS-CoV2.

Methods

Identifying the research question: Is ivermectin effective as a chemoprophylaxis and treatment in COVID-19 patients?

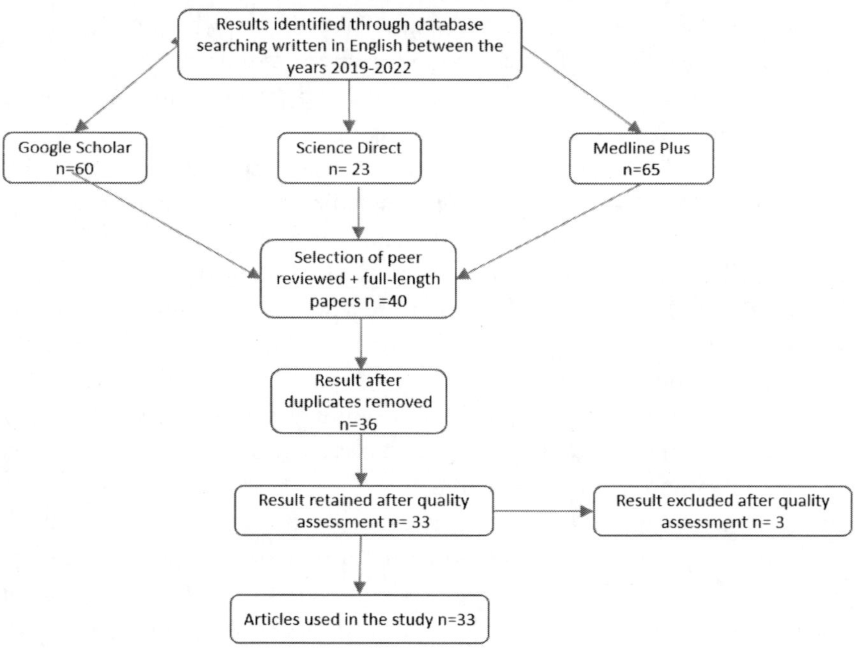

Figure 1. Flow Chart diagram of selecting studies for inclusion in the narrative review.

Search methods for identifying relevant studies: A literature search was conducted with the following Boolean operators "COVID-19 treatment and prophylaxis" or "ivermectin treatment and prophylaxis for COVID-19" or "ivermectin treatment and prophylaxis for SARS- CoV2 infection" on Google Scholar database using the advance setting and then the following other databases of Science Direct and Medline Plus. All articles written in English within the period 2019-2022 were selected. A list of 148 articles was generated from the initial search. The peer-reviewed papers with full text were selected, and the titles and abstracts were studied. Lastly, the quality assessment of the abstracts and the full text of the papers was done, eliminating papers with significant methodological flaws (inappropriate study design for the study aim). Finally, 33 articles were used to write the narrative review paper.

Study selection

Inclusion: Peer-reviewed studies on the effectiveness of ivermectin in the treatment and prophylaxis of COVID-19 patients in Egypt, Argentina, France, Bangladesh, India, Nigeria, Iraq, Spain, and Pakistan between 2019-2022.

Exclusion: Exclusion of short communications, editorials, mini-reviews, book chapters, encyclopedias, one paper was retracted and papers with methodological flaws.

Charting the data, collating, and summarizing: A summary of each paper was written, highlighting the type of paper, sample size, dosage, and frequency of ivermectin use, the location of the study, and the important clinical findings. Both statistically significant and nonsignificant data were recorded. The information was also presented in a table with the different headings of ivermectin prophylaxis trials in COVID-19 patients, ivermectin efficacy in COVID-19 outpatients with mild-moderate disease, and ivermectin efficacy in hospitalized COVID-19 patients. Each heading had the subheading: type of paper, sample size, dosage, frequency of ivermectin use, the location of the study, and the important clinical findings.

Reporting the results: The clinical evidence from the literature review based on the following headings were reported: Summary of ivermectin prophylaxis trials in COVID-19 patients, a summary of ivermectin efficacy in mild-moderate COVID-19 outpatients, and a summary of ivermectin efficacy in hospitalized COVID-19 patients (see Figure 1 above).

Analysis and findings

Summary of the ivermectin prophylaxis trials in COVID-19 patients: two RCTs and five observation studies. Data from two RCTs and five observational studies showed statistically significant decreases in the transmission of COVID-19 among human subjects using ivermectin prophylaxis.

Randomized controlled trials

Shouman et al. (14) conducted an RCT in Egypt by randomized 304 asymptomatic participants (close contacts with COVID-19 patients) either to ivermectin (intervention) or a placebo (control) group. The intervention group received 0.25 mg/kg of ivermectin on the day of the positive test of the index case and after seventy-two hours. The control group did not receive ivermectin. Fifteen patients in the interventional group tested positive for COVID-19 after two weeks versus fifty-nine family members in the control group, 7.4% versus 58.4%, $P < 0.001$ (14).

Another RCT conducted in Argentina (n=234) by Chahla et al. (15) found that healthcare workers in the intervention group received 12 mg of ivermectin weekly, 3.4% contracted COVID-19 versus 21.4% of the controls (receiving placebo), $p < 0.01$.

Observational studies

Alam et al. (16) in Bangladesh performed a prospective observational (OCT) study (n = 118) with the experimental group receiving an oral dose of 12 mg of ivermectin monthly for four months and the control group receiving a placebo.

The difference between the two groups was significantly large, with 6.7% in the experimental group testing positive for COVID-19 vs. 73.3% of subjects in the control group diagnosed with COVID-19 after four months, $P < 0.001$ (16). Even if the study was not blinded, the results were similar to the other RCT trials conducted, making it less likely that confounders alone were the reasons for the observed finding.

Table 1. A summary of the efficacy of Ivermectin use in prophylaxis against COVID-19 disease

Author	Country	Study design	Number of participants	participants	Ivermectin dose	Ivermectin frequency	Outcome reported
Shouman et al. (2021)	Egypt	RCT	340	Two groups of asymptomatic (household) close contacts diagnosed and confirmed with RT-PCR COVID-19 index case. One group received Ivermectin; the other did not. F/u for two weeks for the development of symptoms.	Participants received Ivermectin based on body weight. If body weight was 40–60 kg: 15 mg of Ivermectin was given, 60–80 kg: 18 mg of Ivermectin was given, and > 80 kg: 24 mg was given.	Two doses are given 72 hours apart	Fifteen contacts (7.4%) developed COVID-19 symptoms in the intervention arm compared to 58.4% in the non-intervention arm ($p < 0.001$)
Chahla et al. (2021)	Argentina	RCT	234	Health care workers	12 mg every seven days	Every seven days	The participants diagnosed with COVID-19 in the experimental group were lower, only 4 of 117 (3.4%) than subjects in the control group: 25 of 117 (21.4%) (p-Value = 0.0001)
Carvallo et al. (2020)	Argentina	OCT	229	Asymptomatic health care workers with a negative COVID-19 PCR test	1 drop of Ivermectin (0.6 mg / ml).	Five times a day for 28 days	No health workers treated with IVERCAR tested positive for COVID-19 after 28 days of initial treatment. Eleven healthcare personnel (11.1%) in the comparator group yielded positive swabs ($p < 0.001$).

Author	Country	Study design	Number of participants	participants	Ivermectin dose	Ivermectin frequency	Outcome reported
Carvallo et al. (2020)	Argentina	OCT	1195	Health care workers	12 mg	Once weekly for up to 10 weeks	Zero percent of the 788 workers taking Ivermectin versus fifty-eight percent of the 407 controls contracted COVID-19 ($p < 0.001$).
Bernigaud et al. (2021)	France	OCT	69	Nursing home residents	0.2 mg/kg	Once	Of participants receiving Ivermectin, 10.1% contracted COVID-19 versus 22.6% in the control group. Zero percent (0.0%) mortality in prophylaxis group versus 4.9% in control group ($P < 0.05$).
Alam et al. (2020)	Bangladesh	OCT	118	Health care workers	12 mg	monthly	6.9% of participants in the experimental group contracted COVID-19 versus 73.3% in the control group, $P < 0.05$
Behera et al. (2020)	India	Case-control	186	Health care workers	0.3 mg/kg	Day 1 and day 4	Two doses of Ivermectin on day one and then on day 4 reduced the risk of COVID-19 infection (OR 0.27 95% CI 0.16–0.53) $P < 0.05$.

Carvallo et al. (17) also performed a prospective observational trial on 229 healthy volunteers. One hundred and thirty-one patients were treated with a combination of ivermectin and carrageenan, while the controls took a placebo. None (0%) of those receiving the intervention tested positive for COVID-19 vs. 11.2% of patients in the control arm, p < 0. 001 (17). A more extensive observational prospective study by the same team included 1,195 health care workers (17). Seven hundred and eighty-eight workers received the Ivermectin Carrageenan combination treatment, while the others adhered to standard personal protection equipment. The intervention group took 12 mg of ivermectin weekly. Over three months, there were no infections among the prophylaxis group compared to 58% who became ill with COVID-19 in the controlled group (17). The ivermectin carrageenan combination was separately tested with the RCT by the Ministry of Health in Argentina, summarized above, with statistically significant results. The results showed that 12 mg of ivermectin a month is sufficient to prevent COVID-19 infections among healthcare workers, p < 0.0001 (15).

In a case-control study conducted by Behera et al. (18) involving 372 healthcare workers in India, seventy-seven participants took ivermectin prophylaxis versus controls who took placebos. Health care workers in the interventional arm had a 73% reduction in COVID-19 infection (OR = 0.27, CI 0.15 – 0.51) (18).

In another case-control study conducted by Bernigaud et al. (19), among nursing home residents in France treated with ivermectin for scabies were 69 residents and 52 staff members. Only 10.1% of residents fell ill with COVID-19 during the period surrounding the treatment of scabies, and none died (19). The investigator chose controls from surrounding nursing homes and found that 22.6% of residents fell ill, with 4.9% death (19).

The data reviewed and summarized in Table 1 shows the evidence of ivermectin in prophylaxis studies. The general theme from the two randomized control trials (14, 15) and five observational control trials (16-19) demonstrated large significant statistical reductions in the transmission of COVID-19. It is essential that even if five observational trials were used, the results obtained were similar to the randomized control trials and demonstrated beneficial evidence in human prophylaxis against the COVID-19 disease.

Summary of the efficacy of ivermectin in treating mild-moderately ill COVID-19 outpatients seen in seven randomized controlled trials

An RCT conducted by Mahmud et al. (20) in Bangladesh randomized 363 participants with mild to moderate COVID- 19 symptoms to the intervention (ivermectin plus doxycycline) group versus the control (placebo). Results were statistically significant with increased rates of early improvement with the number of patients with ≤7- day recovery, $P < 0.03$, and decreased clinical deterioration, $P < 0.02$ (20).

Ravikirti et al. (21) performed a double-blinded RCT on 115 patients randomized, with participants in the interventional arm receiving 12 mg of ivermectin on days one and two of admission and participants in the control arm receiving a placebo. The primary outcome testing on PCR positivity for up to six days was not different between groups; however, the mortality was lower in the intervention arm versus the control arm, 0% vs. 6.9%, $P = 0.19$ (21).

Babalola et al. (22) performed an RCT in Nigeria with 62 patients randomized into three groups. The first group received 6 mg of ivermectin twice weekly, and the second group received 12 mg of ivermectin twice weekly. The third group received standard of care treatment plus a placebo. Results were statistically significant in a dose-dependent fashion for viral clearance in low and high-dose treatment groups vs. the control group, $p = 0.006$ (22).

Hashim et al. (23) conducted an RCT in Iraq on 140 COVID-19 patients who were randomized to the ivermectin/doxycycline combination in addition to the standard of care versus the control group receiving the standard treatment only. Time to recovery was statistically significantly shorter in the intervention group vs. the control group, with $P < 0.0001$ (23).

Chaccour et al. (24) conducted a double-blinded RCT in Spain with 24 mildly COVID-19 patients, randomized to receive ivermectin vs. placebo. Results were statistically significant for the decrease in viral load, patient days without smell, and patient days with cough in the treatment group, $P < 0.05$ (24).

In Bangladesh, Chowdhury et al. (25) conducted an RCT on 120 mildly ill COVID-19 patients randomized into ivermectin and doxycycline treatment arm or hydroxychloroquine-Azithromycin in the control arm. The time to recover from symptoms approached statistical significance showing superiority in the treatment group vs. the control group, 5.9 days versus seven days, $p = 0.07$ (25).

Table 2. The efficacy of Ivermectin in treating mild- moderately ill COVID-19 outpatients

Author	Country	Study design	Number of participants	Participants	Ivermectin dose	Ivermectin frequency	Outcome recorded
Mahmud 2020)	Bangladesh	Double-blinded RCT	363	COVID-19 patients with symptoms: Hospitalized and outpatients with mild to moderate COVID-19 illness	12 mg + doxycycline	Once, within three days of the PCR+ test.	60% of participants in the treatment group had a ≤ 7- day recovery vs. 44% in the placebo group, Hazard ratio = 0.06; 95% CI (confidence interval) 0.04-0.09, $P < 0.001$.
Ravikirti et al. (2021)	India	RCT	115	Mild to moderate COVID-19 patients	12 mg	Daily for two days	There was no difference in negative PCR up to day six between the two groups ($P = 0.19$) and no in-hospital mortality in the intervention arm; however, there were four deaths in the placebo arm.
Chowdhury et al. (2021)	Bangladesh	RCT	116	Mild to moderate COVID-19 patients	0.2 mg/kg + doxycycline	Once	The time to symptomatic recovery in the experimental group was 5.9 days versus 9.3 days ($P = 0.07$)
Babalola et al. (2021)	Nigeria	Double-blinded RCT	62	Mild–moderate illness	6 mg and 12 mg	Every two days for a period of two weeks	Time to viral clearance: 4.6 days with a high dose of Ivermectin versus 6.0 days with a low dose of Ivermectin versus 9.1 days in the control group ($P = 0.006$)
Podder et al. (2020)	Bangladesh	RCT	62	Outpatients with mild-moderate COVID-19 illness	0.2 mg/kg	Once	Ivermectin had no beneficial clinical effect on the disease course over the usual standard of care in mild to moderate COVID-19 cases.

Author	Country	Study design	Number of participants	Participants	Ivermectin dose	Ivermectin frequency	Outcome recorded
Hashim et al. (2020)	Iraq	RCT	140	2/3 outpatients and 1/3 hospital patients	0.2 mg/kg + doxycycline	Daily for 2–3 days	Recovery time was 6.3 days in the treatment arm versus 13.6 days in the control arm ($P < 0.001$). 0% in the treatment arm versus 27.3% mortality in the control arm for the severely ill patients ($P = 0.052$).
Chaccour et al. (2021)	Spain	RCT	24	Outpatients	0.4 mg/kg	Once	No diff in PCR positivity on day 7, lower viral load on days 4 and 7, 76 versus 158 patients, $P < 0.05$. Days of anosmia 68 versus 98 patients, $P < 0.05$. Days of cough, $P < 0.05$.

Table 3. Clinical trials of ivermectin in hospitalized patients

Author	Country	Study design	Number of participants	Participants	Ivermectin dose	Ivermectin frequency	Outcome recorded Tx versus control
Niaee et al. (2021)	Research square	RCT	180	Hospitalized patients	0.2,0.3,0.4 mg/kg (3 dosing strategies)	Once vs. days one, two, and three.	Mortality: 3.3% in the intervention arm versus 18.3% in the control arm. OR = 0.18, CI 0.06–0.55, $P < 0.05$.
Hashim et al. (2020)	Iraq	RCT	140	Hospitalized patients	0.2 mg/kg + doxycycline	Daily for 2-3 days	Time to recovery was 6.34 days in the experimental arm versus 13.66 days in the control arm ($P < 0.01$). There was 0% mortality in the treatment arm vs. 27.3% mortality in the control arm in the severely ill patients ($P = 0.052$). The rate of progression to illness in the treatment arm was 9% vs. 31.8% in the control arm ($P = 0.15$).
Ahmed et al. (2021)	Bangladesh (Dhaka)	RCT	72	Hospitalized patients	12 mg	Daily for five days	Virological clearance was earlier in the 5-day Ivermectin treatment arm when compared to the placebo arm (9.7 days vs. 12.7 days; $P = 0.02$)
Chachar et al. (2020)	Pakistan	RCT	50	COVID-19 hospital patients	12 mg	Two doses on day one and one dose on day 2	There was no significant difference in being asymptomatic on day seven at follow-up between the experimental and control groups ($P = 0.5$)

Podder et al. (26) randomized 62 mild to moderately ill COVID-19 patients to a single dose of ivermectin orally (200 mg/kg) in addition to usual care versus the control group receiving usual care only. Time to symptomatic recovery was shorter in the treatment group versus the control group and approached statistical significance, $P > 0.05$ (26).

Table 2 summarizes the evidence of Ivermectin efficacy in mild-moderate COVID-19 patients. Statistically significant reductions in time to recovery and a decrease in length of hospital stay were seen in two randomized control trials, $P < 0.05$ (22, 23), with one with a near statistically significant ($P = 0.07$) decrease in time to recovery by approximately five days (25). Considering the sample size of the RCT done by Chowdhury et al. (25), n = 116, is crucial. Hashim et al. (23) conducted the RCT in Iraq, n = 140, and showed a large reduction in mortality, with 27.3% more patients in the control group dying than in the interventional group. The study also reports a decreased rate of deterioration and hospitalization in COVID-19 patients; however, even with such a large reduction in mortality, the study results were not of statistical significance, $P = 0.052$ (23). It may be possible that if these two studies (23, 25) were repeated in the future with larger sample sizes, they would approach statistical significance. Therefore, recommending a meta-analysis to increase the sample sizes of these and similar studies can give better evidence of the clinical efficacy of ivermectin use. Two RCTs gave evidence of statistically significant reductions in viral load, cough and days of anosmia (24, 27).

Summary findings on the efficacy of ivermectin treatment in COVID-19 hospitalized patients in four RCTs

Hashim et al. (23) conducted an RCT with 140 COVID-19 patients randomized to intervention versus control groups. Both groups included 22 hospitalized patients. The treatment group received ivermectin/doxycycline and included 11 severely ill patients, and 11 critically ill patients, whereas the control group receiving standard of care had only severely ill patients (23). There was a significant reduction in the progression rate to illness (9% vs. 31.8%, $P = 0.15$) and significant differences in mortality among severely ill groups in the treatment arm vs. the control arm, 0% vs. 27.3%, $P = 0.052$ (23). None of these endpoints achieved statistical significance, which could be due to the small sample size. However, time to recovery was statistically significant with 6.34 days in the experimental arm versus 13.66 days in the control arm, $P < 0.01$ (23).

Niaee et al. (28) conducted an RCT in Iran with 180 participants randomized to multiple ivermectin dosing versus the control group receiving the standard of care treatment with a placebo. The average mortality was 3.3% in the treatment arm versus 18.8% in the standard of care and placebo arm, OR of 0.18, 95% CI of 0.06 – 0.55, $P < 0.05$ (28).

An RCT conducted in Bangladesh by Amhed et al. (27) randomized 72 hospitalized COVID-19 patients in multiple groups. The first group received 12 mg of oral ivermectin for five days; the second group received a combination of ivermectin and doxycycline for four days, and the third group received a placebo. Results were statistically insignificant between the three groups for the mean length of hospital stay after treatment ($p = 0.93$) (27).

In an RCT conducted in Pakistan by Chachar et al. (29), fifty participants were randomly assigned to either the intervention group receiving ivermectin and symptomatic treatment or the control group only receiving symptomatic treatment. There was no statistically significant difference in those asymptomatic at seven days, $p = 0.5$ (29).

Table 3 summarizes the efficacy of ivermectin in hospitalized COVID-19 patients. one RCTs showed large statistically significant evidence in the reduction of mortality in hospitalized patients (28). Chachar et al. (29) conducted an RCT on fifty patients and failed to demonstrate significant findings of being asymptomatic after seven days of treatment with ivermectin, $P = 0.5$. The study may not have shown significant findings due to the low sample size or the patient's mild COVID-19 infections.

To date, the evidence-based efficacy of ivermectin against the COVID-19 disease is overwhelming. Ivermectin is a safe drug with few adverse side effects (9) and has both antiviral and anti-inflammatory properties (7,8). Caly et al. (10) showed that ivermectin inhibits the replication of SARS- CoV2 by various proposed mechanisms. Two molecular studies later showed that ivermectin inhibits the SARS- CoV2 entry into host cells (11,30). Ivermectin is clinically beneficial in chemoprophylaxis (15, 16) and was reported to significantly reduce viral load (24, 27). In addition, ivermectin decreased the transmission and clinical deterioration in mild to moderately ill COVID-19 patients (23) and decreased the mortality in severely ill patients (28).

Table 4 shows the differences in the methods of 12 studies. Most studies describe randomization using a computerized random process (20-22, 24, 27-29) whereas five studies fail to use random sequence generation for randomization, introducing selection bias (14, 15, 23, 25, 26). Selection bias is also introduced because of the lack of allocation concealment in five studies (14, 15, 23, 25, 26). The risk of performance bias because of the failure to blind the participants and detection bias due to the failure to blind the investigators were seen in 3 studies (23, 26, 29). On the other hand, double blinding was seen in two RCTs (20, 22).

Apart from the differences in study methods, the difference in the effective prophylaxis dose and frequency must be emphasized. The large observational study conducted by Carvallo et al. (17) in Argentina showed that 12 mg of ivermectin weekly for up to ten weeks could be used as prophylaxis against COVID-19. However, Chahla et al. (15), in a randomized clinical trial in collaboration with the Ministry of Health in Argentina, suggested that 12 mg of ivermectin monthly for ten months is sufficient for prophylaxis. Other major differences in the study's design, participant recruited and characteristics, ivermectin dosage and frequency, and outcomes recorded for the prophylaxis, mild-moderately ill COVID-19 patients, and severely ill COVID-19 patients can be found in Tables 1-3 above.

Table 4. Comparison of the study design of the studies used. Differences between study methods

Studies	Random sequence generation	Allocation concealment	Blinding of participants	Blinding of investigators
Ahmed et al. (2021)	yes	yes	uncertain	uncertain
Babalola et al. (2021)	yes	yes	yes	yes
Chaccour et al. (2021)	yes	yes	yes	uncertain
Chachar et al. (2020)	yes	uncertain	No	No
Chahla et al. (2021)	No	No	No	uncertain
Chowdhury et al. (2021)	No	No	No	uncertain
Hashim et al. (2020)	No	No	No	No
Mahmud (2020)	yes	yes	yes	yes
Niaee et al. (2021)	yes	yes	uncertain	uncertain
Podder (2020)	No	No	No	No
Ravikirti et al. (2021)	yes	yes	yes	uncertain
Shouman et al. (2021)	No	No	uncertain	uncertain

Gaps

One study failed to fully describe allocation concealment (29), and three studies failed to describe the blinding of the participants in the method (14, 27, 28). In addition, it was uncertain in seven studies whether investigators were blinded (14, 15, 21, 24, 25, 27, 28) making it difficult and challenging to analyze and assess biases. Furthermore, the authors whose methods were unclear and lacked full descriptions should be contacted for more information on the studies since there are limited RCTs on ivermectin treatment in COVID-19 patients.

Limitations

Firstly, some studies used ivermectin as the intervention and compared it to the standard of care (23, 25) or a placebo (20). The narrative review did not subgroup or analyze the studies based on ivermectin doses or whether the controls received standard care or placebo. Variation in the dose of ivermectin use and whether ivermectin was compared to a placebo, or the standard of care makes it difficult to assess the effectiveness of ivermectin.

Secondly, most studies have a small sample size (19, 24). Studies of ivermectin are newly repurposed against the COVID-19 disease, with existing trials suggesting conflicting results and no evidence from meta-analysis supporting ivermectin efficacy (9). Therefore, getting consent from patients to sign up for the studies may be difficult.

Thirdly, failure to document or perform randomization, allocation concealment, and blinding in some studies introduces bias and decreases the quality of studies (14, 15, 23).

Fourthly, the lack of a meta-analysis to determine the pooled effect of ivermectin use for COVID-19 patients and the lack of treatment guidelines from governing health authorities. The challenges faced by health care providers in deciding the best therapeutic interventions for COVID-19 patients would be significantly reduced if more evidence-based medicine guidelines came from the governing health authorities (9).

Conclusion

Ivermectin is a safe, orally taken, widely available drug with antiviral properties against SARS-CoV2 replication and entry into the host cells. The drug is also clinically beneficial in chemoprophylaxis and treatment of COVID-19 patients with various disease severity. Despite this, the need for more quality and quantity of data and meta-analysis for public health agencies to give therapeutic guidance and recommendations on using ivermectin in the chemoprophylaxis and treatment of COVID-19 patients even in a growing pandemic. In addition, more funding is needed to conduct more RCTs globally with large sample sizes on ivermectin's ability in the efficacy and chemoprophylaxis of the COVID-19 disease.

References

[1] Crump A, Ōmura S. Ivermectin, 'Wonder drug' from Japan: the human use perspective. Proc Jpn Acad 2011;87(2):13-28.

[2] Colson P, Raoult D. Fighting viruses with antibiotics: an overlooked path. Int J Antimicrob Agents 2016;48(4):349–52.

[3] Trivedi N, Verma A, Kumar D. Possible treatment and strategies for COVID-19: review and assessment. Eur Rev Med Pharmacol Sci 2020;24(23):12593-608.

[4] Babalola OE. Ocular onchocerciasis: current management and prospects. Clin Ophthalmol 2011; 5:1479–91.

[5] Padhy BM, Mohanty RR, Das S, Meher BR. Therapeutic potential of Ivermectin as add-on treatment in COVID-19: A systematic review and meta-analysis. J Pharm Pharm Sci 2020; 23:462–9.

[6] Santin AD, Scheim DE, McCullough PA, Yagisawa M, Borody TJ. Ivermectin: A multifaceted drug of Nobel prize-honored distinction with indicated efficacy against a new global scourge, COVID-19. New Microbes New Infect 2021;43:100924.

[7] Chan W, He B, Wang X, He ML. Pandemic COVID-19: Current status and challenges of antiviral therapies. Genes Dis 2020;7(4):502–19.

[8] Rizzo E. Ivermectin, antiviral properties, and COVID-19: A possible new mechanism of action. Naunyn Schmiedebergs Arch Pharmacol 2020;393(7):1153-6.

[9] Kory P, Meduri GU, Varon J, Iglesias J, Marik PE. Review of the emerging evidence demonstrating the efficacy of ivermectin in the prophylaxis and treatment of COVID-19. Am J Ther 2021;28(3):e299–318.

[10] Caly L, Druce JD, Catton MG, Jans DA, Wagstaff KM. The FDA-approved drug Ivermectin inhibits the replication of SARS-CoV-2 in vitro. Antiviral Res 2020;178: 104787.

[11] Bryant A, Lawrie TA, Dowswell T, Fordham EJ, Mitchell S, Hill SR, Tham TC. Ivermectin for prevention and treatment of COVID-19 infection: A systematic review, meta-analysis, and trial sequential analysis to inform clinical guidelines. Am J Ther 2021;28(4):434-60.

[12] Lehrer S, Rheinstein PH. Ivermectin docks to the SARS-CoV-2 spike receptor-binding domain attached to ACE2. In Vivo 2020;34(5):3023–6.

[13] Gudadappanavar AM, Benni J. An evidence-based systematic review on emerging therapeutic and preventive strategies to treat novel coronavirus (SARS-CoV-2) during an outbreak scenario. J Basic Clin Physiol Pharmacol 2020;31(6). doi: 10.1515/jbcpp-2020-0113.

[14] Shoumann WM, Abdelmonem AH, Nafae RM, Ragab MI, Samra SR, Dalia AI, et al. Use of ivermectin as a potential chemoprophylaxis for COVID-19 in Egypt: A randomized clinical trial. J Clin Diagnostic Res 2021;15(2):27–32.
[15] Chahla RE, Medina Ruiz L, Ortega ES, Morales RN, Marcelo FB, George A, et al. Intensive treatment with ivermectin and iota-carrageenan as pre-exposure prophylaxis for COVID-19 in health care workers from Tucuman, Argentina. Am J Ther 2021;28(5):e601–4.
[16] Alam MT, Murshed R, Bhiuyan E, Saber S, Alam RF, Robin RC. A case series of 100 COVID-19-positive patients treated with the combination of ivermectin and doxycycline. J Bangladesh Coll Phys Surg 2020;38:10–5.
[17] Carvallo H, Roberto HG, Psaltis AJ, Veronica CO. Study of efficacy and safety of topical ivermectin + iota-carrageenan in the prophylaxis against COVID-19 in health personnel. J Biomed Res Clin Investig 2020;2(1):1-6.
[18] Behera P, Patro BK, Singh AK, Chandanshive PD, Ravikumar SR, Pradhan SK, et al. Role of Ivermectin in preventing COVID-19 infection among healthcare workers in India: A matched case-control study. PLoS One 2021;16(2):e0247163.
[19] Bernigaud C, Guillemot D, Ahmed-Belkacem A, Grimaldi-Bensouda L, Lespine A, Berry F, et al. Oral ivermectin for a scabies outbreak in a long-term care facility: potential value in preventing COVID-19 and associated mortality. Br J Dermatol 2021;184(6):1207-9.
[20] Mahmud R. A randomized, double-blind, placebo-controlled clinical trial of ivermectin plus doxycycline for the treatment of confirmed Covid-19 infection. Dhaka: Dhaka Medical College (Bangladesh) 2020. URL:https://www.clinicaltrials.gov/ProvidedDocs/31/NCT04523831/Prot_ICF_000.pdf.
[21] Ravikirti X, Roy R, Pattadar C, Raj R, Agarwal N, Biswas B, Manjhi PK, et al. Evaluation of ivermectin as a potential treatment for mild to moderate COVID-19: A double-blind randomized placebo controlled trial in Eastern India. J Pharm Pharmaceut Sci 2021;24:343-50.
[22] Babalola OE, Bode CO, Ajayi AA, Alakaloko FM, Akase IE, Otrofanowei E, et al. Ivermectin shows clinical benefits in mild to moderate COVID19: a randomized controlled, double-blind, dose-response study in Lagos. QJM 2021;114(11):780-8.
[23] Hashim HA, Maulood MF, Rasheed AM, Fatak DF, Kabah KK, Abdulamir AS. Controlled randomized clinical trial on using Ivermectin with Doxycycline for treating COVID-19 patients in Baghdad, Iraq. Iraqi J Med Sci 2021;19(1):107-15.
[24] Chaccour C, Casellas A, Blanco-Di Matteo A, Pineda I, Fernandez-Montero A, Ruiz-Castillo P, et al. The effect of early treatment with ivermectin on viral load, symptoms and humoral response in patients with non-severe COVID-19: A pilot, double-blind, placebo-controlled, randomized clinical trial. EclinicalMedicine 2021;32:100720.
[25] Chowdhury TA, Shahbaz M, Karim R, Islam J, Guo D, He S. A comparative study on ivermectin-doxycycline and hydroxychloroquine-azithromycin therapy on COVID-19 patients. Eurasian J Med Oncol 2021;5(1):63-70.
[26] Podder CS, Chowdhury N, Sina MI, Haque WMMU. Outcome of ivermectin treated mild to moderate COVID-19 cases: A single-center, open-label, randomized controlled study. IMC J Med Sci 2020;14(2):11-8.

[27] Ahmed S, Karim MM, Ross AG, Hossain MS, Clemens JD, Sumiya MK, et al. A five-day course of ivermectin for the treatment of COVID-19 may reduce the duration of the illness. Int J Infect Dis 2021;103:214–6.

[28] Niaee MS, Namdar P, Allami A, Zolghadr L, Javadi A, Karampour A, et al. Ivermectin as an adjunct treatment for hospitalized adult COVID-19 patients: A randomized multicenter clinical trial. Asian Pac J Trop Med 2021;14(6):266-73.

[29] Chachar AZK, Khan KA, Asif M, Tanveer K, Khaqan A, Basri R. Effectiveness of ivermectin in SARS-CoV-2/COVID-19 patients. Int J Sci 2020;9:31-35.

[30] Ramezani Z, Dayer MR, Noorizadeh S, Thompson M. Deactivation of SARS-CoV-2 via shielding of spike glycoprotein using carbon quantum dots: Bioinformatics perspective. COVID 2021;1(1):120-9.

Chapter 9

Prostate cancer incidences and survival by race: A narrative review

Krishna Thakore, MD, MPH
Anthony La, BA
Deepak Kumar Palanichami, BSc
Osazee Eguagie, MD, PGCME
Victor Adedara, BSc, MS
Abidemi Fasanmi, MD, MPH, PhD
Marios Loukas, MD, PhD
and Emmanuel O Keku*, MD, MA, MSPH, FRSPH, FAHA
School of Medicine, Department of Public Health and Preventive Medicine,
St George's University, St George, Grenada, West Indies

Abstract

Prostate cancer is the most common form of newly diagnosed cancers in men in the United States. Understanding the trends in prostate cancer incidence and survival among various racial groups can potentially help us guide prevention strategies and screening guidelines for at-risk populations. Demographic and clinical data on prostate cancer patients' incidence and survival was obtained from SEER public-use data set.

* Corresponding Author's Email: ekeku@sgu.edu; Emmanuel O Keku, MD, MA, MSPH, Professor and Track Director, MD/MPH program, School of Medicine, St George's University, Department of Public Health, and Preventive Medicine, POBox 7, St George, Grenada, West Indies.

In: Public Health
Editors: Emmanuel O Keku and Joav Merrick
ISBN: 979-8-89113-083-8

Prostate cancer survival rates were acquired by computing relative survival for the SEER-identified prostate cancer patients. Additionally, a literature search was performed using PubMed and Google Scholar to explore non-modifiable risk factors and other lifestyle factors affecting the incidence and survival of prostate cancer. Prostate cancer incidence has drastically increased since the introduction of PSA in 1988 and subsequently, approved by USFDA in 1994. The 5-year mortality for prostate cancer was higher in African American men than in Caucasians. High-fat diet, smoking, and obesity showed association with increased risk of prostate cancer incidence and worse prognosis. Prostate cancer affects African American men more than Caucasian men with a lower relevant survival rate. African American men between the age of 55 to 69 could benefit from routine PSA screening.

Keywords: prostate cancer, incidence, survival, trends, mortality, race, African American, racial disparity, lifestyle factors, obesity, smoking

Introduction

Prostate cancer is the most common form of newly diagnosed cancer in men over the age of 65 years with 21% of all estimated new cancer cases in 2020 in the United States (US) (1). Additionally, prostate cancer is the second most common cause of cancer death with 10% of all estimated cancer deaths in 2020 among men in the US (1). The probability of developing prostate cancer in a man's lifetime is 1 in 9 (2). The risk factors for prostate cancer include age, family history, genetics, race and lifestyle. This study examines a large cohort of prostate cancer patients in the US with efforts to identify demographics like races that impact clinical outcomes. Understanding the trends in prostate cancer incidence and survival among various racial groups can potentially help us guide prevention strategies and screening strategies for at-risk populations.

Prostate specific antigen (PSA), digital rectal examination and transrectal ultrasound-guided biopsy have been used clinically for more than two decades to diagnose prostate cancer (3). PSA screening has allowed not only for early detection and treatment of prostate cancer, but also a reduction in prostate-specific death rates. Since 1986 when PSA screening was first introduced in the US and approved by the United States Food and Drug Administration (USFDA) in 1994, more than a million additional men have been diagnosed with and treated for prostate cancer, the majority at early stages (4-7). The current guideline for PSA screening for men aged 55 to 69 years is Class C (individual decision) and Class D (do not screen) for men aged 70 years and above (6). The goal of this study is to extract the incidence and survival data for prostate cancer for different races and review literature to find modifiable and non-modifiable risk factors to provide supporting evidence for PSA screening recommendations based on race as well as individualized lifestyle risk factors.

Methods

The National Cancer Institute's (NCI) Surveillance, Epidemiology, and End Results (SEER) database was used to find the incidence of prostate cancer and 5-year relative survival data. The SEER 18 database includes 27.8% of the US population, including 24.9% of the total Caucasian population, 25.6% of the total African American population, 30.6% of the total American Indian/Alaska Native population, 38.4% of the total Hispanic population, 50.4% of the total Asian population, 66.5% of total Native Hawaiian/Pacific Islander population and 43.7% of the total population of other races.

Using the SEER*Stat software (version 8.3.8), the incidence of prostate cancer from 1973 to 2015 was generated by using the inclusion criteria of ICD-0-3 site recode- Prostate, age at diagnosis- 55 years and older (5, 8). The incidence data were further stratified by race to obtain the proportion of new cases among different races by adding inclusion criteria of each race in the SEER*Stat software. Additionally, the 5-year relative survival of prostate cancer by race was calculated by the Kaplan-Meier method in SEER*Stat (5, 8). The relative survival was calculated in SEER*Stat software by dividing the overall survival for prostate cancer patient to the overall survival for similar cancer-free population (9). The non-cancer patients from populations were derived from life tables matching by age, sex, and race, and patients were stratified by age, race, and year of diagnosis (9). The incidence of prostate cancer and relative survival rates were graphically obtained using Microsoft Excel.

To further explore the risk factors in prostate cancer incidence and survival, a literature search was conducted on Google Scholar and PubMed databases between January 1970 and February 2021 using the following keywords with Boolean operators: Prostate cancer, incidence, survival, risk factors, racial disparity, prognosis, African American, lifestyle factors, obesity and smoking.

Results

A total of 1,161,654 patients were identified in SEER as satisfying the entrance criteria for prostate cancer incidence between 1973 to 2015 (see Table 1). Incidence of prostate cancer in 5-year interval was drastically increased from 1988 after the introduction of PSA screening and furthermore after 1994 following the USFDA approval of PSA screening test (see Figure 1). The incidence trends continued to increase until 2007 after which it stabilized over the 5-year period (see Figure 1). The incidence stratification by race shows about 80% of cases in Caucasian and about 13% of cases in African American among the population included in the SEER database (see Table 1).

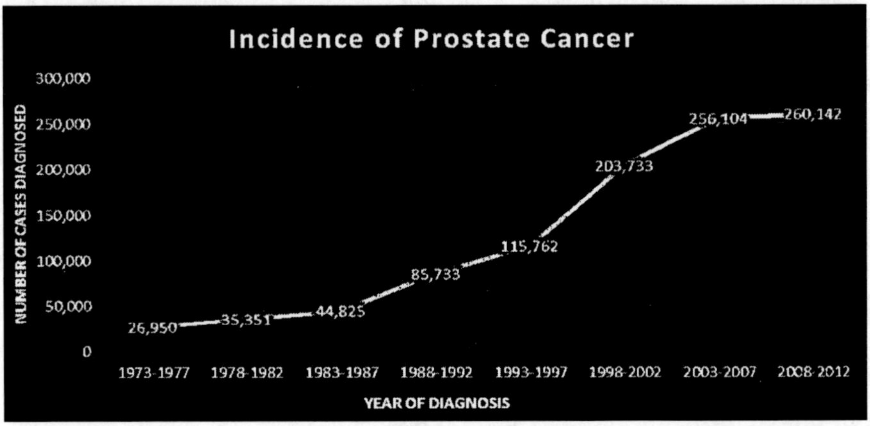

Figure 1. Incidence of prostate cancer (SEER 18: 1973-2012).

Table 1. Prostate cancer incidence by race (SEER 18: 1973-2015)

Race	New Cases	Percentage
Caucasian	935,417	80.52%
African American	147,274	12.68%
American Indian/Alaska Native	3,930	0.34%
Asian or Pacific Islander	53,362	4.59%
Unknown	21,671	1.87%
Total	1,161,654	100%

Prostate cancer 5-year relative survival was lower in African American men than Caucasian men between the years 2000 to 2015 (see Table 2). The 5-year relative survival for African American men is 95.99% while Caucasian men had relative survival of 98.92%. Among other races, American Indian/Alaska Native had the lowest 5-year relative survival of 94.67% and

Asian or Pacific Islander had relative survival of 95.63% (see Table 2, Figure 2).

The relative survival for American Indian/Alaska native was the lowest, although the sample size of American Indian/Alaska Native is much lower than other races (see Table 2). The literature review highlights some of the important risk factors of prostate cancer and can help us modify the screening guidelines for prostate cancer. The major risk factors for prostate cancer are increasing age, race, genetic factors, and family history (2, 4). The risk of prostate cancer for men aged 60 to 69 years is 1 in 21, while the risk increases to 1 in 12 for men 70 years and older (2). The incidence of prostate cancer is about 60% higher in men of African descent than Caucasian in the US and the Caribbean (2). Furthermore, African American men have worse prognosis of prostate cancer with lower relative survival than Caucasian men (see Table 2, Figure 2). Probable reasons behind the disparity could be due to differences in treatments offered for prostate cancer or lifestyle factors including diet and obesity.

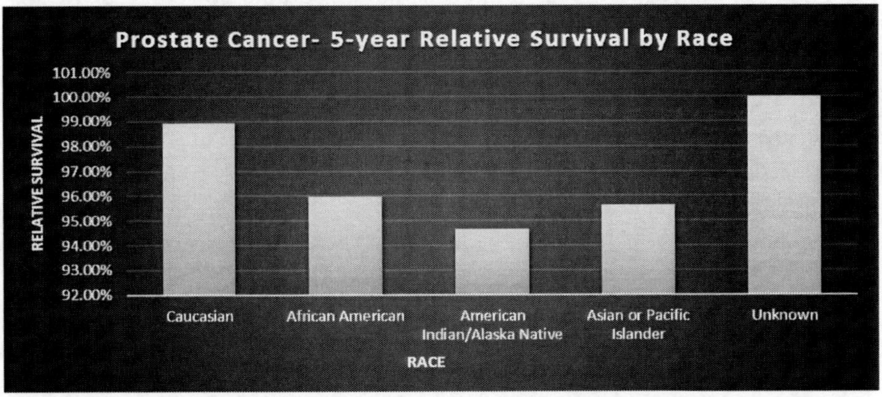

Figure 2. Prostate cancer 5-year relative survival by race (SEER 18: 2000-2015).

Table 2. Prostate cancer 5-year relative survival by race (SEER 18: 2000-2015)

Race	Number of cases	Relative Survival
Caucasian	563,256	98.92%
African American	99,274	95.99%
American Indian/Alaska Native	2,557	94.67%
Asian or Pacific Islander	35,065	95.63%
Unknown	17,089	100.00%

Discussion

Since the introduction of PSA screening in 1988, there has been a steady increase in relative survival of prostate cancer patients (10). This may be the result of over-diagnosis or lead time bias after the PSA era (10). Due to the controversial nature of PSA screening in overdiagnosis and overtreatment of prostate cancer with small to no reduction in prostate cancer- specific mortality, USPSTF updated their recommendation for PSA screening to Class D (do not screen) for men of all ages in 2012 (6, 7, 11, 12). However, most recent guidelines from USPSTF in 2018 recommend Grade C (individual decision) for men aged 55 to 69 years, due to recent higher incidence in metastatic prostate cancer in men without PSA screening (6, 7, 11). Since the current guideline is Grade C for PSA screening, all men aged 55 to 69 years are not routinely screened by their healthcare providers. Recently, Sharma et al. (13) showed that recent increase in metastatic prostate cancer can be explained by reduction in PSA screening in recent years. Additionally, based on the current epidemiological trends in incidence and survival, Rawla (4) predicted that there will be an 80% increase in incidence of prostate cancer by 2040. The highest incident increase is predicted in Africa with 120% increase, followed by Latin American and Caribbean with 101% by 2040 (4). Considering higher incidence rate and lower relative survival rate, all men of African descent over the age of 55 years could benefit from routine screening with PSA.

Increasing age is a well-established risk factor for prostate cancer (2). Current USPSTF guidelines recommend Grade D (do not Screen) for men aged 70 years and older (6). Huynh-Le et al. (2020), performed a cross-sectional study among men diagnosed with prostate cancer in Norway and showed that increased age is significantly associated with more invasive disease (14). Based on this study, after considering individual risk factors, older men aged 70 years and above might benefit from PSA screening rather than not being screened at all (14). Some research has found that elderly cancer patients are more likely than younger ones to positively change their health behaviors after a cancer diagnosis, especially smoking cessation (15).

Other significant modifiable lifestyle risk factors include obesity, diet, and smoking (4). Allott et al. (16), showed that obesity is associated with advanced prostate cancer and increased risk of prostate cancer treatment failure. Fujita et al. (17), hypothesized that an increased inflammatory state caused by obesity plays a role in prostate cancer growth due to local changes in the immune cells of adipose tissue. Based on these studies, losing weight might be beneficial in reducing the risk of aggressive prostate cancer as well as in the management of prostate cancer (17). Narita et al. (18), showed that a high-fat diet increases the risk of prostate cancer by possible growth factor signaling, inflammation, metabolism, and hormonal modulation which is also consistent with the risk of obesity. On the other hand, foods containing vitamin E, calcium, omega-3 fatty acids, zinc, beta-carotene, and selenium have a potential protective effect on the risk of prostate cancer (19). Thus, the incorporation of more plant-based foods and fish may help with reducing the risk of prostate cancer (19).

Smoking is a well-established risk for various cancers of epithelial cell origin and heart disease. In a prospective study, Kenfield et al. (20) showed that smoking at the time of diagnosis increases the risk of overall mortality and prostate cancer-specific mortality as well as recurrence. Additionally, smoking cessation for 10 years showed similar prostate cancer mortality as non-smokers (20). Smoking cessation counseling can be beneficial to both avoid prostate cancer and reduce mortality among patients with a diagnosis of prostate cancer (21).

Bhardwaj et al. (22) explored the molecular causes of racial disparity among higher incidence and mortality for prostate cancer among men of African descent. Bhardwaj et al. (22) found that diet, environmental factors, and lifestyle factors impact susceptible genetics among African men negatively. Additionally, the risk associated with obesity is higher in African American men for high-grade prostate cancer (23). In addition to epigenetic factors, men of African descent face a longer wait time between the diagnosis of prostate cancer and treatment as compared to Caucasian men (24). Odedina et al. (25), showed a high burden of prostate cancer among African American men of West African ancestry that follows the path of the Transatlantic Slave Trade. However, Benjamins et al. (26), conducted a population study in 50 US cities to compare African American and Caucasian mortalities among men living in the same city and found that the mortality in African American was significantly higher than Caucasian patients due to the disparity in availability of care between the two races. Moreover, men of African descent also have higher incidence of prostate cancer in the age group of less than 50 years old as compared to Caucasian men (27).

Strength

This study shows the trends in incidence of prostate cancer among all races since the introduction of PSA as a screening test in the US. Furthermore, it also shows survival trends showing higher mortality in African American men diagnosed with prostate cancer. The discussion explores the modifiable and non-modifiable risk factors through a literature review and current screening recommendations. The survival data by race along with evidence from literature can help us set up screening guidelines based on race instead of a universal screening guideline for prostate cancer for all ethnicities.

Limitations

This study does not have incident rates among different races. The total population for each race was not available for specific SEER databases. However, the incidence rates were included by race from literature review and meta-analysis data for data analysis and discussion. Lifestyle risk factors such as smoking, diet, and obesity have been shown to increase the risk of prostate cancer leading to an associated worse prognosis. However, more research is needed to provide clear underlying pathophysiology of each lifestyle risk factor.

Conclusion

Race plays a significant role in the incidence and survival of prostate cancer. African American men aged 55 to 69 years could benefit from regular PSA screening for earlier diagnosis and treatment. Additionally, African American men over 70 years old and younger than 50 years old should be considered for PSA screening based on their individualized family history, obesity and other lifestyle risk factors.

References

[1] Siegel RL, Miller KD, Jemal A. Cancer statistics, 2020. CA Cancer J Clin 2020;70(1):7-30.

[2] Tarver T. Cancer facts and figures 2012. American Cancer Society (ACS). J Consum Health Internet 2012;16(3):366-7.
[3] Smart R. PSA testing and DRE, TRUS scanning with sector biopsy, improved histology, curative treatments, and active surveillance for prostate cancer: a success story for men's health. NZ Med J 2008;121(1287):57–68.
[4] Rawla P. Epidemiology of prostate cancer. World J Oncol 2019;10(2):63–89.
[5] Surveillance, Epidemiology, and End Results (SEER) Program (www.seer.cancer.gov) SEER*Stat Database: Incidence - SEER 18 Regs Custom Data (with additional treatment fields), Nov 2017 Sub (1973-2015 varying) - Linked To County Attributes - Total U.S., 1969-2016 Counties, National Cancer Institute, DCCPS, Surveillance Research Program, released April 2018, based on the November 2017 submission.
[6] Schröder FH, Hugosson J, Roobol MJ, Tammela TLJ, Ciatto S, Nelen V, et al. Screening and prostate-cancer mortality in a randomized European study. N Engl J Med 2009;360(13):1320–8.
[7] Eastham J. Prostate cancer screening. Investig Clin Urol 2017;58(4):217–9.
[8] Surveillance, Epidemiology, and End Results (SEER) Program. SEER*Stat Database: Incidence - SEER Research Data, 18 Registries, 2019. URL: www. seer. cancer. Gov.
[9] Mariotto AB, Noone AM, Howlader N, Cho H, Keel GE, Garshell J, et al. Cancer survival: An overview of measures, uses, and interpretation. J Natl Cancer Inst Monogr 2014;2014(49):145-86.
[10] Draisma G, Boer R, Otto SJ, van der Cruijsen IW, Damhuis RA, Schröder FH, et al. Lead times and overdetection due to prostate-specific antigen screening: estimates from the European Randomized Study of Screening for Prostate Cancer. J Natl Cancer Inst 2003;95(12):868–78.
[11] Grossman DC, Curry SJ, Owens DK, Bibbins-Domingo K, Caughey AB, Davidson KW, et al. Screening for prostate cancer: US Preventive Services Task Force Recommendation Statement. JAMA 2018;319(18):1901–13.
[12] Lin K, Croswell JM, Koenig H, Lam C, Maltz A. Prostate-specific antigen-based screening for prostate cancer: An evidence update for the US Preventive Services Task Force. Rockville, MD: Agency for Healthcare Research and Quality, Report 12-05160-EF-1, 2011.
[13] Sharma V, Venkataramana A, Comulada WS, Litwin M, Saigal C. Association of reductions in PSA screening across states with increased metastatic prostate cancer in the United States. J Clin Oncol 2021;39(6):228.
[14] Huynh-Le MP, Myklebust TA, Feng CH, Karunamuni R, Johannesen TB, Dale AM, et al. Age dependence of modern clinical risk groups for localized prostate cancer—A population-based study. Cancer 2020;126(8):1691–9.
[15] Niu C, Eng L, Qiu X, Shen X, Espin-Garcia O, Song Y, et al. Lifestyle behaviors in elderly cancer survivors: A comparison with middle-age cancer survivors. J Oncol Pract 2015;11(4):e450–9.
[16] Allott EH, Masko EM, Freedland SJ. Obesity and prostate cancer: Weighing the evidence. Eur Urology 2013;63(5):800–9.

[17] Fujita K, Hayashi T, Matsushita M, Uemura M, Nonomura N. Obesity, inflammation, and prostate cancer. J Clin Med 2019;8(2):201.

[18] Narita S, Nara T, Sato H, Koizumi A, Huang M, Inoue T, et al. Research evidence on high-fat diet-induced prostate cancer development and progression. J Clin Med 2019;8(5):597.

[19] Chan JM, Gann PH, Giovannucci EL. Role of diet in prostate cancer development and progression. J Clin Oncol 2005;23(32):8152–60.

[20] Kenfield SA, Stampfer MJ, Chan JM, Giovannucci E. Smoking and prostate cancer survival and recurrence. JAMA 2011;305(24):2548–55.

[21] De Nunzio C, Andriole GL, Thompson IM Jr, Freedland SJ. Smoking and prostate cancer: A systematic review. Eur Urol Focus 2015;1(1):28–38.

[22] Bhardwaj A, Srivastava SK, Khan MA, Prajapati VK, Singh S, Carter JE, et al. Racial disparities in prostate cancer: A molecular perspective. Front Biosci (Landmark Ed) 2017;22(5):772–82.

[23] Pietro GD, Chornokur G, Kumar NB, Davis C, Park JY. Racial differences in the diagnosis and treatment of prostate cancer. Int Neurourol J 2016;20(Suppl 2):S112–9.

[24] Kinlock BL, Thorpe RJJ, Howard DL, Bowie JV, Ross LE, Fakunle DO, et al. Racial disparity in time between first diagnosis and initial treatment of prostate cancer. Cancer Control 2016;23(1):47–51.

[25] Odedina FT, Akinremi TO, Chinegwundoh F, Roberts R, Yu D, Reams RR, et al. Prostate cancer disparities in Black men of African descent: a comparative literature review of prostate cancer burden among Black men in the United States, Caribbean, United Kingdom, and West Africa. Infect Agent Cancer 2009;4(Suppl 1):S2.

[26] Benjamins MR, Hunt BR, Raleigh SM, Hirschtick JL, Hughes MM. Racial disparities in prostate cancer mortality in the 50 largest US cities. Cancer Epidemiol 2016;44:125–31.

[27] Parker PM, Rice KR, Sterbis JR, Chen Y, Cullen J, McLeod DG, et al. Prostate cancer in men less than the age of 50: A comparison of race and outcomes. Urology 2011;78(1):110–5.

Chapter 10

HIV infection disparities in Louisiana: Directions for primary care providers

Monica Edward, MD, MPH, CCFP
Anthony La, BA
Deepak Kumar Palanichami, BSc
Temiloluwa Ogunmoyin, BSc
Azeez Kuteyi, BScN
Abidemi Fasanmi, MD, MPH, PhD
and Emmanuel O Keku*, MD, MA, MSPH
School of Medicine, Department of Public Health and Preventive Medicine, St George's University, St George, Grenada, West Indies

Abstract

Louisiana is suffering from an epidemic of HIV, and East Baton Rouge has been listed as one of the jumpstart locations for the CDC's priority programs to end HIV. The populations that are disproportionately impacted are gay, bisexual, and other men who have sex with men (GBM), those who identify as transgender, and minorities. This narrative review is aimed to understand why these populations experience HIV disproportionately. Condom use, pre-exposure prophylaxis (PrEP) access and use, race, ethnicity, sexual orientation, and incarceration were found to be major contributors. Primary care practitioners (PCPs) are a vital part of the next steps to address these shortcomings by providing HIV primary care. This would be embodied by providing sensitive and

* Corresponding Author's Email: ekeku@sgu.edu.

In: Public Health
Editors: Emmanuel O Keku and Joav Merrick
ISBN: 979-8-89113-083-8

unbiased care, prescribing PrEP, prescribing antiretroviral medications, and incorporating more holistic care. This holistic care could involve workshops for HIV education, practice negotiating condom use, and working with a multidisciplinary team to decrease sociodemographic disparities. Furthermore, PCPs can act as the healthcare bridge between incarceration and post-release. There was no literature regarding transgender populations in Louisiana. This is an important direction for future research.

Keywords: human immunodeficiency virus, HIV, people living with HIV, PLWH, acquired immunodeficiency syndrome, AIDS, gay, bisexual, men who have sex with men, GBM, minority, transgender, incarceration, pre-exposure prophylaxis, PrEP, primary care provider, PCP, Louisiana

Introduction

Human immunodeficiency virus (HIV) has moved from being a disease predominantly found in urban gay communities to an epidemic impacting the Southern United States (US) (1). Despite only making up 28% of the entire US population, southern states accounted for 51% of new HIV diagnoses in the US and dependent areas (1,2). The states considered the "deep South," which are the most impacted, include: Alabama, Florida, Georgia, Louisiana, Mississippi, North Carolina, South Carolina, Tennessee and Texas.

Among large metropolitan areas in the US, Louisiana, with an HIV case rate of 20.9 per 100,000 population, ranked fourth in the US for HIV case rates in 2018 with Baton Rouge and New Orleans ranking third and seventh, respectively (3). East Baton Rouge Parish has been named one of the jumpstart priority areas of the ending the HIV epidemic by the Health and Human Services agencies (1). Among those diagnosed with HIV in Louisiana, the highest HIV infection rates and HIV-related mortality has been found in men who have sex with men (GBM), Black, and transgender persons (3). Blacks accounted for 70% of newly diagnosed HIV cases and 72% of newly diagnosed AIDS (acquired immunodeficiency syndrome) cases despite only making up 32% of Louisiana's population. GBM constituted 57% of new HIV diagnoses – the majority of whom were black (68%). These discrepancies are due to several factors including race, stigma, lack of social support, poverty, isolation, incarceration, and inequitable care within the healthcare system. Additionally, HIV infection rates have increased among transgender persons in the South, especially for those who are transgender male-to-female and among those who are Black/African American (4).

HIV is a preventable disease, and progression to AIDS is also preventable with consistent use of antiretrovirals (ARVs). Without intervention, there will be increased HIV transmission and infection rates, increased healthcare dollars spent for complications of HIV and AIDS, increased AIDS-related mortality, and worsening health status for already marginalized individuals. In this narrative review, the research question that was asked was: why are there disparities in HIV infection amongst Black, GBM, and transgender persons in Louisiana?

Methods

This review involved an appraisal of articles of an epidemiological, medical, and social science nature. Data sources included the CDC HIV/AIDS Surveillance Report for 2018 and the State of Louisiana Department of Health 2018 STD/HIV Surveillance Report. In addition, there was a comprehensive literature search on the topic of HIV in Louisiana using PubMed and Scopus. The MeSH terms HIV, AIDS, Louisiana, black, gay, MSM (male sex with male), transgender, disparity, incarceration, and primary care were used.

Study selection

The search resulted in a total of 107 articles. English language articles on the human species that were published between 2011 and 2021, with full text available were included. The articles that were found to be conference proceedings, pre-publication stage articles, protocol publications, or studies with children less than 12 years of age were excluded. Titles and abstracts were reviewed and only those articles that involved the population of interest were included in the final review. A summary of these 15 articles can be found in Table 1. There were no articles found that focused on transgender populations.

Results

The majority of new HIV diagnoses in 2018 were among GBM – with 68% of new diagnoses in black men and 69% under the age of 35 years (3). Consistent condom use and PrEP use are especially important to prevent HIV transmission among GBM. Unfortunately, there has been limited uptake of PrEP with two independent national studies approximating that 4% of GBM used pre-exposure prophylaxis (PrEP) (5). It is estimated that in 2019, there were 77 PrEP users per 100,000 of the population in Louisiana, with most of the users identifying as male or between the ages of 25-34 years (6). The PrEP-to-Need Ratio was found to be 2.38 in those aged 13-24 years indicating unmet needs as compared to any other age group.

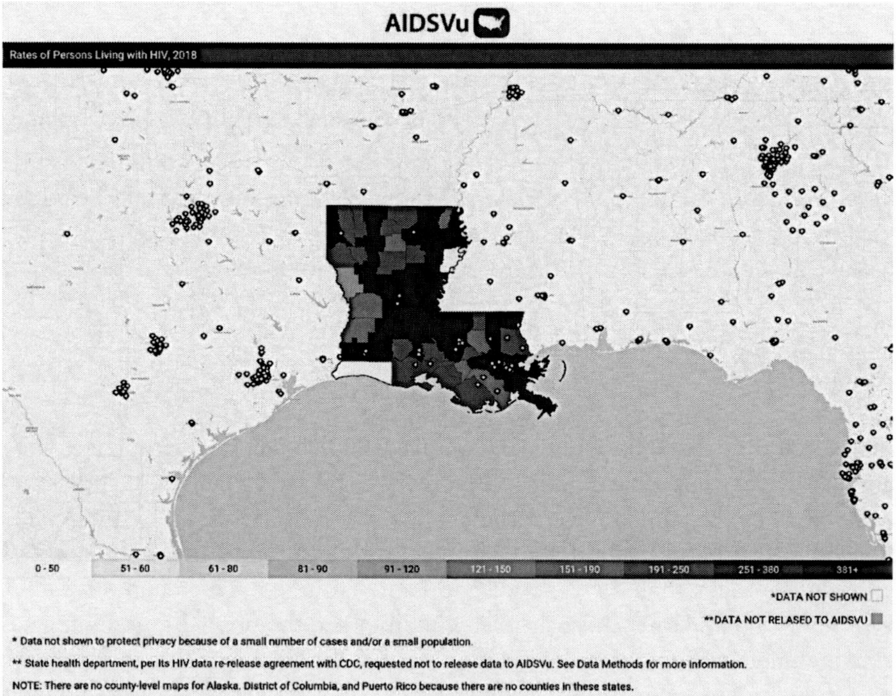

Figure 1. Map of Louisiana counties. Each county is shaded according to rates of PLWH as of 2018 (legend just below the map). Overlay of locations with PrEP services available as of March 2021. This map is demonstrating that the majority of PrEP service locations can be found in New Orleans and Baton Rouge leaving many other areas with high rates of PLWH with either no services or too few services (6).

Table 1. Summarized analysis of articles found in PubMed and Scopus during literature review

Article Title	Authors	Study Design	Publication Date	Summary
HIV Prevention Interventions to Reduce Racial Disparities in the United States: A Systematic Review	Hemmige, McFadden, Cook, Tang, and Schneider	Systematic Review	2012	There were no studies specifically aimed to reduce HIV incidence or risk behaviour between various racial/ethnic groups. They also found that few interventions used HIV incidence as a primary endpoint or targeted GBM populations. Successful interventions measuring behavioural change involved actively teaching skills to initiate and maintain behavioural change rather than passive, didactic teaching.
Understanding Structural Barriers to Accessing HIV	Levy, Wilton, Phillips II, Glick,	Literature review	2014	Racism and homophobia during healthcare visits, and a lack of social support from

Table 1. (Continued)

Testing and Prevention Services Among Black Men Who Have Sex with Men (BMSM) in the United States	Kuo, Brewer, Elliott, Watson , and Magnus			social networks limit comprehensive HIV testing and prevention services. Positive patient-provider relationships decrease risk behaviours, increase condom use, increase HIV testing, decrease number of sexual partners, and increase frequency of asking for a partner's HIV status prior to engaging in intercourse. There is a lack of access to healthcare services due to lack of insurance coverage, high perceived costs-benefit analysis of healthcare, and frequent contact with the prison system which results in inconsistent access to HIV prevention.
Elevated Sexual Risk Behaviours Among Postincarcerated Young	Ricks, Crosby, and Terrell	Randomized Control Trial	2015	Men with a previous history of incarceration were more likely to use alcohol before sex, were high while having

African American Males in the South				sex, and were more likely to want to conceive a pregnancy. Men who were previously incarcerated were less likely to use a condom during their last sexual encounter, were more likely to exchange sex for drugs or money, and were less likely to have had sex with a male partner in the last 2 months. After controlling for individual socioeconomic factors, prior incarceration was correlated with and predicted risky sexual behaviours. Incarceration history was also a predictor for risky sexual behaviour even after controlling for the intervention group.
Understanding Structural Barriers to accessing HIV	Levy, Wilton, Phillips II, Glick,	Literature review	2014	Black MSM are less likely than other MSM to disclose their sexual behaviour or identity

Table 1. (Continued)

Testing and Prevention Services Among Black Men Who Have Sex with Men (BMSM) in the United States	Kuo, Brewer, Elliott, Watson, and Magnus			to physicians due to concerns around confidentiality, discrimination, distrust, comfort, and conspiracy theories. PrEP implementation is limited due to the unwillingness of physicians to prescribe it. Barriers to ART adherence and retention in care among Black MSM living with HIV include medical miscommunication, mistrust, racism, low levels of healthcare provider cultural competency, and sexual prejudice. Stigma, discrimination, incarceration, and poverty also impact black MSM living with HIV.
Mass incarceration and the impact of prison release on	Ojikutu, Srinivasan, Bogart,	Cross sectional study	2018	Baton Rouge had the highest median 5-year HIV diagnosis rate of all the cities. HIV diagnosis rate was moderately associated

HIV diagnoses in the US South	Subramanian, and Mayer			with prison release rate and prison release rate was moderately associated with percent population living in poverty and percent non-Hispanic Black population. Baton Rouge had the strongest correlation of prison release rate with overall, male and female HIV diagnosis rate. Males are incarcerated at higher rates than females, have higher HIV diagnosis rates, and that prison release was significantly associated with male HIV diagnosis rate.
HIV, Sexually Transmitted Infection, and Substance Use Continuum of Care Interventions Among Criminal Justice-Involved Black Men	Harawa, Brewer, Buckman, Ramani, Khanna, Fujimoto, Schneider	Systematic Review	2018	There were no studies on transgender individuals. The intervention types that were found were mostly around education or condom provision, HIV and STI screening, harm reduction, or modeling.

Table 1. (Continued)

Who Have Sex with Men: A Systematic Review				Most interventions were focused on screening and linking PLWH to care. They found that HIV and STI education was the most common focus of HIV prevention in this population. Condom distribution, prevention skill building, needle exchange, and treatment as prevention interventions were rare or nonexistent. PrEP was not described in any studies. Black MSM were rarely direct targets of focused interventions while incarcerated and transgender women were nonexistent.
Racial Discrimination and HIV-related Risk Behaviors in Southeast Louisiana	Kaplan, Hormes, Wallace, Rountree, and Theall	Cross-sectional, secondary analysis	2016	Experiences of discrimination were significantly associated with lifetime history of STIs and sexual risk taking. Alcohol use

				was not a mediatory between history of STIs or sexual risk and discrimination.
Participation in community groups increases the likelihood of PrEP awareness: New Orleans NHBS-MSM Cycle, 2014	Ransome, Zarwell, and Robinson	Cross sectional study	2019	The authors hypothesized that GBM who report more participation and trust in community groups will have higher likelihoods of being aware of and willing to use PrEP. 47% of GBM were aware of PrEP however there was not a statistically significant willingness to use PrEP in these groups. The authors suggested that this may be due to structural barriers or stigma. Interestingly, being 40 years of age or older was significantly associated with willingness to use PrEP.

Table 1. (Continued)

Network Properties Among Gay, Bisexual and Other Men Who Have Sex with Men Vary by Race	Zarwell and Robinson	Cross sectional study	2019	This study sought to investigate variations in social and sexual network properties among Black and White GBM in New Orleans. Black participants were younger, reported fewer risk behaviours, had less social support, were less likely to frequent gay venues, and had networks with fewer members they could talk to.
Correlates of Durable Viral Suppression (DVS) Among Criminal Justice-involved (CJI) Black Men Living with HIV in Louisiana	Brewer, Issema, Moore, Chrestman, Mukherjee, Odlum, and Schneider	Secondary data analysis	2019	Those who had no viral suppression and some viral suppression were more likely to have lived with HIV for longer and less likely to be adherent at baseline. The group with some viral suppression was less likely to have received an HIV-related service during their last incarceration and more likely to report being severely depressed.

Implementation of a Socio-structural Demonstration Project to Improve HIV Outcomes Among Young Black Men in the Deep South	Brewer, Daunis, Ebaady, Wilton, Chrestman, Mukherjee, Moore, Corrigan, and Schneider	Prospective longitudinal study	2019	This report aimed to describe the background, rationale, intervention, and results of the Louisiana Integrated Center for Care, Supportive Services, and Community Health. Almost half of participants living with HIV achieved viral suppression with client-centred care coordination interventions. Housing discrimination based on sexual orientation and race occurs and is covert in nature.
PrEP Indicators, Social Capital, and Social Group Memberships among Gay, Bisexual, and Other Men Who Have Sex with Men	Zarwell, Ransome, Barak, Gruber, and Robinson	Cross sectional study	2019	This study looked at social group memberships as a possible marker of social capital. They found that community group participation was associated with PrEP awareness. Those who belonged to social groups in addition to their chosen families

Table 1. (Continued)

				were over 10 times as likely to be aware of PrEP. Younger ages and higher education were associated with PrEP willingness.
HIV prescriptions on the frontlines: Primary care providers' use of antiretrovirals for prevention in the Southeast United States, 2017	Henny, Duke, Buchacz, Brooks, Samandari, and Sutton	Cross sectional study	2020	The authors of this study examined data from the Knowledge, behaviours, Attitudes, and Practices of HIV-Related Care among healthcare providers in high HIV burden areas of the Southeast. Overall there were low levels of prescribing PrEP and ART. They found that providers who were familiar with one type of preventative ARV were likely to prescribe other preventative ARVs. The number of PCPs that ever prescribed PrEP or ARVs was low.

Using Financial Incentives to Improve Rates of Viral Suppression and Engagement in Care of Patients Receiving HIV Care at 3 Health Clinics in Louisiana: The Health Models Program, 2013-2016	Brantley, Burgess, Bickham, Wendell, and Gruber	Prospective cohort study	2018	This study discussed the findings from the first few years of a Health Models program that provided financial incentive for meeting certain performance measures to improve rates of HIV care engagement and viral suppression at 3 clinics in New Orleans and Baton Rouge. The number of patients who were virally suppressed after 12 months of enrollment in the program increased from 57.8% to 82.7%. Transgender females, young patients, MSM, Hispanics/Latinos, patients diagnosed <1 year at baseline, patients with annual income <$15,000, and those not taking ART at baseline had the largest increases in rates of viral suppression. Furthermore,

Table 1. (Continued)

				96.3% of patients with at least 12 or 24 months of follow-up data had continued in care between 12 and 24 months of enrollment.
An exploratory study of resilience, HIV-related stigma, and HIV care outcomes among men who have sex with men (MSM) living with HIV in Louisiana	Brewer, Hood, Moore, Spieldenner, Daunis, Mukherjee, Smith-Davis, Brown, Bowen, and Schneider	Prospective cohort study	2020	There was a positive association between resilience and HIV care outcomes in a majority Black MSM population. Black MSM living with HIV experienced HIV-related stigma resulting in healthcare interruptions. Black MSM experienced greater consequences of HIV stigma and had poorer outcomes. They also found that having higher levels of resilience is associated with less time since last HIV care visit especially for Black MSM.

PrEP awareness among the GBM community is high, with approximately 90% of men hearing about PrEP; however, only 28.8% of those men have reported PrEP use in the last year (3). This is especially the case among GBM who belong to a community group as they were more likely to be aware of PrEP and agreeable to use it compared to those who were not (7). Low uptake has been attributed to factors such as financial barriers, lack of social support, stigma, conspiracy beliefs, and location of clinics, as seen in Figure 1 (5).

The responsibility for PrEP use does not just fall on the patient, but also on the provider. In a recent study of ARV prescriptions in the Southeast US for either PrEP, non-occupational post-exposure prophylaxis (nPEP), or highly active antiretroviral therapy, researchers found that 81.9% of providers had never prescribed PrEP and 52.1% of providers responded that they "know little about it/never heard of it" (8). The authors found that PrEP prescriptions were associated with a higher degree of familiarity among providers. This is problematic when so many providers are not familiar with it – resulting in only 18.1% of PCPs ever prescribing PrEP.

Race, ethnicity and sexual orientation

Race and ethnicity, especially for those identifying as African American, are notable risk factors for subpar medical treatment in PLWH (9). Several factors contribute to this including poorer access to healthcare and social services, lack of trust in the healthcare system, stigma, poverty, unstable housing, higher rates of incarceration, and belief that homosexuality is morally wrong (9,10). Discrimination based on race is unfortunately common in Louisiana, with one study reporting that African American participants experienced discrimination on more than 34 separate occasions, especially when at school and when receiving services (11). The participants who experienced discrimination were more likely to report risky sexual behaviors, have an increased lifetime history of sexually transmitted infections (STIs), and were less motivated to learn about or access HIV prevention services (11, 12).

Sexual orientation is also a significant risk factor for HIV infection. One study in New Orleans looked at risk factors for new HIV infection and found that being GBM was the leading factor (5). Another study went so far as to compare the prevalence of HIV among Black GBM in this area to the most severely affected regions globally (13). Factors contributing to this are likely unprotected receptive anal intercourse and smaller sexual networks. Black MSM living with HIV are more likely to have a detectable viral load, more likely to have a lower CD4 count, and more likely to have comorbid STIs than their non-Latino White MSM counterparts, which consequentially increases HIV transmission risk (12). Furthermore, Black MSM experiencing a greater impact of enacted HIV stigma were less likely to have accessed HIV care or completed labs within the last year (14). On the other hand, those MSM who had an undetectable viral load were more likely to report high levels of resiliency.

Incarceration

Louisiana has a prison incarceration rate of 680 per 100,000, the highest in the US compared with the national average of 419 per 100,000 (15). While Black individuals make up 32% of the total population in Louisiana, they make up approximately 60% of the individuals incarcerated (16). This is a consequence of the introduction of harsher drug laws in the 1970s. This resulted in more arrests, guilty sentences, and incarceration of drug users in poor, metropolitan areas. This is compounded by policies for habitual offenders with misdemeanors, longer minimum sentences, and limited employment prospects resulting in higher rates of reoffending and incarceration.

Testing for HIV on entering or while in prison is only conducted in 20 states, and only three states test prisoners before their release (12). In 2015, of those in custody in Louisiana, 3.4% had HIV (17). Louisiana has an opt-out process for HIV testing during intake and only tested if requested by an offender or if pre-parole testing was required upon discharge. Louisiana also does not offer HIV testing during routine medical exams while incarcerated, but only if it is a high-risk group, when requested by the prisoner, when clinically indicated, when the court ordered, or after involvement in an incident. It was noted that regular HIV testing was only offered by 5 out of 104 parish jails due to the cost of ARVs, lack of Medicaid coverage for incarcerated persons, and limited availability of Ryan White Act services for those imprisoned (18). Moreover, while incarcerated, PLWH may experience interruptions in their ARV treatment due to barriers to access to HIV medical services (3).

Upon release, these inmates are also not linked to care services in their home communities which is critical as they are at high risk for risky sexual behaviors when faced with food and housing needs in areas with limited economic opportunities (16). In two separate studies, only 30% of PLWH released from prison filled a prescription for ARVs within 60 days of release and only 28% were registered in care within 90 days (16). One study found that Baton Rouge had the strongest association between release from prison, and the rate of HIV diagnosis, pointing to challenges in the parish or possibly even the state (16). However, recent reports described state-wide issues in carrying out HIV testing, administering ARVs, and discharge planning.

Incarceration is a structural risk factor that has been associated with HIV transmission. It has been found that when groups of men are compared, those previously incarcerated are 3-6 times more likely to be infected with HIV (12, 19). One study on young African American men aged 15-23 years old found that previously incarcerated men were more likely to use alcohol before sex, be high during sex, engage in unprotected sex, and exchange sexual services for drugs or money (19). These behaviors increase the risk of HIV transmission and infection. Even when controlling for age, age at sexual debut, level of education, level of income, marital status, and housing status, there was a high correlation between a preceding history of incarceration and risky sexual behaviors.

Discussion

To decrease HIV transmission and infection, there needs to be consistent ARV use in PLWH (to achieve undetectable viral loads), consistent condom use, consistent PrEP use, and increased HIV testing. Based on the findings of this review, GBM and Black/African American individuals disproportionately experience HIV infection due to lack of PrEP use, discrimination, inadequate medical care, and high rates of incarceration. PCPs are in the ideal position to address the lack of HIV prevention, testing, and treatment in these areas. Comprehensive primary care clinics can address all the critical areas to reduce HIV transmission and ensure undetectable viral loads for those PLWH in Louisiana. There is increasing evidence that regular contact with healthcare workers may provide greater opportunities to diagnose, treat, and educate about comorbid conditions, such as HIV (20).

If PCPs receive sensitivity training and learn how to navigate conversations about sexual orientation, sexual practices, and HIV in a sensitive manner, there could be less perceived stigma and discrimination. A positive patient-provider relationship can in turn increase condom use, decrease risk behaviors, increase testing, and decrease the number of sexual partners (12). One study found that MSM who shared their sexual behavior or identity with their PCP were more likely to have a positive relationship that facilitated HIV testing and preventative services (12). If PCPs can ensure that they address and acknowledge that Black MSM living with HIV experience challenges related to ARV adherence and retention in care due to factors like mistrust, racism, and poor levels of provider cultural competency, PCPs would make efforts to ensure their patients feel more comfortable. This, type of intervention, can result in better ARV adherence, lower viral loads, and higher CD4 counts. Subsequently, this results in *treatment as prevention* for the spread of HIV among these communities.

PCPs can also address barriers regarding HIV service locations. PCPs can be found all over the state of Louisiana, but as demonstrated in Figures 1 and 2, the locations for HIV testing and PrEP services are not. If more PCPs are willing to become familiar with PrEP and ARV prescribing, they could provide more HIV primary care. This could take the form of HIV education, discussion around sexual practices, sexual orientation, HIV testing, and treatment. Alternatively, there could be more coordinated efforts between infectious disease specialists and PCPs in order to increase PrEP and ARV use. This could potentially result in decreased HIV transmission, decreased HIV infection, and improved rates of viral suppression.

PrEP and condom use are of paramount importance in the prevention of HIV transmission. Interventions that incorporate skills-based teaching instead of knowledge-based approaches are most effective and superior to those using passive learning at reducing sexual risk behaviors in MSM (21). Skills-based training in proper condom use and the practice of negotiating condom use with a sexual partner have been found to increase abstinence, decrease the number of sexual partners and increase condom use for those adolescents nearing the age of sexual debut (22). One systematic review looking for programs that reduced HIV infection among minorities found only a single program that targeted African American GBM (22). This four-session design significantly decreased the proportion of men who had unprotected anal intercourse at the three months follow-up point. This group also found that after training Latino peer leaders in safe sex behaviors, there was an increase in the proportion of persons practicing protected anal intercourse among Latino migrant MSMs after two years.

Utilization of peers or minority health workers (i.e., Black, Latino, MSM) leads to customization of interventions and can increase the acceptance of the behavioral change that is being recommended (22). This is especially true for adolescents. If there are more minority PCPs, nurses, social workers, and peer support workers leading holistic team-based care, there could be better PrEP use, condom use, HIV testing, and retention in care. This would be an interesting aspect to study, one meta-analysis found that "health-worker-based interventions were more efficacious [than peer-based interventions], but that effective interventions were more likely to match health-worker ethnicity with that of the target audience" (22).

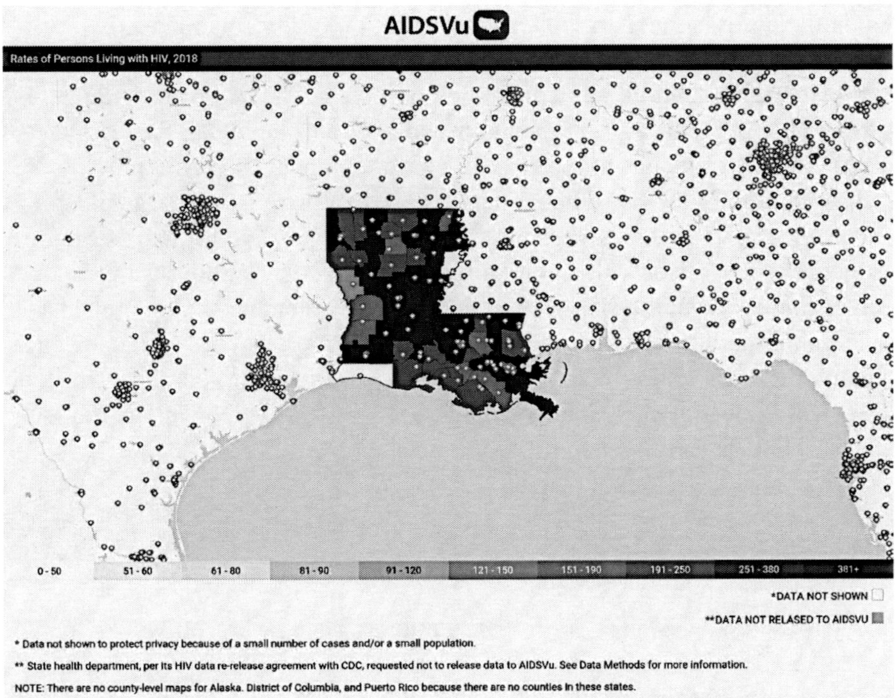

Figure 2. Map of Louisiana counties. Each county is shaded according to the rate of PLWH as of 2018 (legend just below the map). Overlap of locations with HIV testing services. The map demonstrates that most counties have at least 1 HIV testing site for the entire county. Certain counties with urban centers that have higher rates of PLWH have a higher density of testing sites (such as those around New Orleans and Baton Rouge) whereas rural sites with higher rates of PLWH have only 1 testing site for the entire county which can pose a barrier to being tested (6).

Social capital is a critical social determinant in HIV prevention for the GBM community. Having peer-led groups that work closely with a PCP could also have a positive impact on GBM communities. Sexual and social network connections standardize individual health behaviors and can foster healthy or risky behavior which ultimately can dictate individual risk (13). As an example, these networks may comprise families who are not blood relatives due to rejection from their original families. Previous studies found that young

Black GBM who associated with these networks were more likely to report PrEP awareness, having health insurance, and having a PCP (13). Moreover, the volunteer peers within these networks can promote HIV education, prevention, testing, and counseling. The network characteristics should be taken into account as they may influence stigma, social perceptions and standards, access to resources, and dissemination of information (13).

As previously discussed, incarcerated settings are an important area where HIV testing, prevention, and education can occur. The use of programs that involve HIV prevention case managers and peer educators has been shown to increase HIV knowledge and decrease risk behaviors (12). Furthermore, some studies point to improved clinical outcomes when there is discharge planning before release (16). This is a crucial area where PCPs could form a continuous bridge between prison and community HIV care that could ensure regular conversations around HIV testing and ARV adherence. Comprehensive sociodemographic interventions are necessary to improve HIV outcomes. Pre-release education, employment assistance, housing stability, and peer testers and/or counselors are just some examples of areas that can be integrated with clinics to improve HIV outcomes in Louisiana (23).

Limitations

This narrative review has several limitations. There were only two search engines used and only 15 articles were included in the final review making it a small study. This review did not address all populations impacted by HIV in Louisiana, such as IV drug users, women, children under 12 years of age, and perinatal HIV infection. There was also no literature found that addressed the reasons why transgender individuals are disproportionately impacted by HIV in Louisiana. This is an important area for future research as this population has historically been marginalized.

Public health implications

Integration of HIV care into primary care should be a priority to reduce the risk of HIV transmission and infection for GBM, incarcerated males, and Black/African American individuals in Louisiana. These populations experience marginalization and would benefit from non-discriminatory comprehensive care that is preventative from the standpoint of PrEP, condom use, ARV treatment as prevention, HIV testing, and ongoing coordination of care. This approach could potentially reduce HIV transmission and infection in a population that is already struggling with an HIV burden of epidemic proportions.

References

[1] Centers for Disease Control and Prevention. HIV in the Southern United States. United States: NCHHSTP Division of HIV/AIDS Prevention, 2019 September. URL: https://www.cdc.gov/hiv/pdf/policies/cdc-hiv-in-the-south-issue-brief.pdf.

[2] Centers for Disease Control and Prevention. HIV surveillance report, 2020 vol 33. URL: http://www.cdc..gov/hiv/library/reports/hiv-surveillance.html.

[3] State of Louisiana Department of Health. 2018 STD/HIV surveillance report. New Orleans, LA: Louisiana Department of Health, 2018. URL: https://ldh.la.gov/assets/oph/HIVSTD/2018_STDHIV_SurveillanceReport_Final.pdf.

[4] Centers for Disease Control and Prevention. HIV surveillance report, 2019 vol 32. URL: http://www.cdc.gov/hiv/library/reports/hiv-surveillance.html.

[5] Ransome Y, Zarwell M, Robinson WT. Participation in community groups increases the likelihood of PrEP awareness: New Orleans NHBS-MSM Cycle, 2014. PLoS One 2019;14(3):e0213022.

[6] AIDSVu. Local Data: Louisiana. 2018. URL: https://aidsvu.org/local-data/united-states/south/louisiana/.

[7] Zarwell M, Ransome Y, Barak N, Gruber D, Robinson WT. PrEP indicators, social capital, and social group memberships among gay, bisexual, and other men who have sex with men. Cult Health Sex 2019;21(12):1349–66.

[8] Henny KD, Duke CC, Buchacz K, Brooks JT, Samandari T, Sutton MY. HIV prescriptions on the frontlines: Primary care providers' use of antiretrovirals for prevention in the Southeast United States, 2017. Prev Med 2020;130:105875.

[9] Whetten K, Reif S. Overview: HIV/AIDS in the deep South region of the United States. AIDS Care 2007;18(Suppl 1):1–5.

[10] Reif SS, Whetten K, Wilson ER, Mcallaster C, Pence BW, Legrand S, et al. HIV/AIDS in the Southern USA: A disproportionate epidemic. AIDS Care 2013;26(3):351–9.

[11] Kaplan KC, Hormes JM, Wallace M, Rountree M, Theall KP. Racial discrimination and HIV-related risk behaviors in Southeast Louisiana. Am J Health Behav 2016:40(1):132–43.

[12] Levy ME, Wilton L, Phillips G, Glick SN, Kuo I, Brewer RA, et al. Understanding structural barriers to accessing HIV testing and prevention services among Black men who have sex with men (BMSM) in the United States. AIDS Behav 2014;18(5):972–96.

[13] Zarwell M, Robinson WT. Network properties among gay, bisexual and other men who have sex with men vary by race. AIDS Behav 2019;23:1315–25.

[14] Brewer R, Hood KB, Moore M, Spieldenner A, Daunis C, Mukherjee S, et al. An exploratory study of resilience, HIV-related stigma, and HIV care outcomes among men who have sex with men (MSM) living with HIV in Louisiana. AIDS Behav 2022;24(7):2119–29.

[15] The Sentencing Project. State-by-State data, 2020. URL: https://www.sentencingproject.org/the-facts/#detail?state1Option=U.S.Total&state2Option=Louisiana.

[16] Ojikutu BO, Srinivasan S, Bogart LM, Subramanian SV, Mayer KH. Mass incarceration and the impact of prison release on HIV diagnoses in the US South. PLoS One 2018;13(6):e0198258.

[17] Maruschak LM, Bronson J. HIV in prisons, 2015 - Statistical tables. Washington, DC: HIV in Prisons and Jails, 2017. Report No NCJ Number 250641. URL: https://bjs.ojp.gov/library/publications/hiv-prisons-2015-statistical-tables#additional-details-0.

[18] Tarnowski B. Paying the price failure to deliver HIV services in Louisiana Parish jails. New York: Humans Rights Watch, 2016. Report ISBN: 978-1-6231-33375. URL: https://www.hrw.org/report/2016/03/29/paying-price/failure-deliver-hiv-services-louisiana-parish-jails.

[19] Ricks JM, Crosby RA, Terrell I. Elevated sexual risk behaviors among postincarcerated young African American males in the South. Am J Mens Health 2014;9(2):132–8.

[20] Brewer R, Issema R, Moore M, Chrestman S, Mukherjee S, Odlum M, et al. Correlates of durable viral suppression (DVS) among criminal Jjustice-involved (CJI) Black men living with HIV in Louisiana. AIDS Behav 2019;23:2980–91.

[21] Harawa NT, Brewer R, Buckman V, Ramani S, Khanna A, Fujimoto K, et al. HIV, sexually transmitted infection, and substance use continuum of care interventions among criminal justice-involved Black men who have sex with men: A systematic review. Am J Public Health 2018;108(S4):e1–9.

[22] Hemmige V, Mcfadden R, Cook S, Tang H, Schneider JA. HIV prevention interventions to reduce racial disparities in the United States: A systematic review. J Gen Intern Med 2012;27(8):1047–67.

[23] Brewer R, Daunis C, Ebaady S, Wilton L, Chrestman S, Mukherjee S, et al. Implementation of a socio-structural demonstration project to improve HIV outcomes among young Black men in the deep South. J Racial Ethn Health Disparities 2019;6:775–89.

Chapter 11

Elective surgical procedures in the COVID-19 era

Kevin Palmer, MD, MPH
Victor Adedara, BSc, MS
Temiloluwa Ogunmoyin, BSc
Azeez Kuteyi, BScN
Deepak Kumar Palanichami, BSc
Anthony La, BA
Lauren Orlando, PhD
Abidemi Fasanmi, MD, MPH, PhD
and Emmanuel O Keku*, MD, MA, MSPH

School of Medicine, Department of Public Health and Preventive Medicine, St George's University, St George, Grenada, West Indies

Abstract

The coronavirus disease of 2019 (COVID-19) pandemic has altered methods of healthcare delivery which have led to a reduction in the utilization of non-emergent surgical services and a shift towards telehealth. The present study consists of a narrative review of the existing literature which describes the impact of delayed or otherwise altered delivery of surgical services during the COVID-19 pandemic. A review of the PubMed database was conducted utilizing the following search terms: "elective surgery," "COVID," "complications," "delays,"

* Corresponding Author's Email: ekeku@sgu.edu.

In: Public Health
Editors: Emmanuel O Keku and Joav Merrick
ISBN: 979-8-89113-083-8

"hospital delays," "disparity," "social determinants of health," and "equity." The focus of this search was to identify studies and publications related to trends and changes in the delivery of elective surgical services that have resulted, either directly or indirectly because of the COVID-19 pandemic. 114 publications were identified in the search results, and 61 publications were selected for review. These 61 publications were reviewed, analyzed, and the findings are reported under six headings: Definition of elective surgery; Reduction in elective surgical services during the COVID-19 pandemic; Burden of delayed services; Ethical considerations; Moving forward; Further recommendations. The COVID-19 pandemic led to a drastic reduction in elective surgical services. Delays in surgical services and direct complications caused by COVID-19 infection have led to increased morbidity. Implications and recommendations for future practice of telemedicine, and the use of outpatient and same-day surgery centers to avoid spreading COVID-19 infection is, therefore, of great importance.

Keywords: elective surgery, COVID, complications, delays, hospital delays, disparity, social determinants of health, equity

Introduction

The coronavirus disease of 2019 (COVID-19) pandemic has drastically altered methods of healthcare delivery. Efforts to reduce the spread of COVID-19 have been manifested in the form of decreased overall utilization of healthcare services (1), as well as a massive shift towards telehealth services (2, 3). Patients in need of surgical services during the COVID-19 pandemic have faced unique challenges concerning receiving timely and adequate surgical care. Operative procedures have been exclusively limited to those procedures that are deemed emergent in nature (4). This exclusivity is not without justification considering the high transmissibility of COVID-19 (5), which places both patients and healthcare workers at risk of infection. Additionally, perioperative COVID-19 infection is associated with significant postoperative complications and increased mortality rates (6).

With these considerations in mind, the World Health Organization (WHO) issued recommendations and precautions for operative procedures, while also emphasizing that essential surgical treatment should not be neglected (7). Scholarly authors have attempted to objectively define those surgical procedures considered to be "essential." Lackey et al. (8) discussed "nonelective cases" as those "conditions that are life- or limb-threatening or a delay in surgery that will negatively affect the outcome" (p. 60). In the wake of COVID-19, elective cases have been reduced by up to 22% by some estimates (9), while other studies documented surgery reductions of up to 90% with a backlog of surgeries that would take an estimated eight months to resolve in non-pandemic conditions (9).

While the benefit of postponing elective procedures to diminish the spread of COVID-19 is clear (10), the negative consequences of said postponements are not well-defined. Studies have identified the negative psychosocial impact of delaying elective surgical procedures (11, 12, 13). Johnson et al. (14) went on to recognize that certain negative consequences of delayed elective surgical procedures during COVID-19 were disproportionately experienced by non-white patients. The present paper will consist of a narrative literature review with the objective of synthesizing and assessing existing research regarding the negative consequences of the delay of surgical procedures due to the COVID-19 pandemic.

Methods

A review of the literature was conducted utilizing the PubMed database. Searches were conducted utilizing the varying combinations of the following search terms: "elective surgery," "COVID," "complications," "delays," "hospital delays," "disparity," "social determinants of health," and "equity." The focus of these searches was to identify studies and publications related to trends and changes in the delivery of elective surgical services that have resulted, either directly or indirectly because of the COVID-19 pandemic. To include a wide scope of studies, and publications a broad and open interpretation of the causative and correlative relationships between the COVID-19 pandemic and any associated changes in the delivery of surgical services were included. As this is a narrative review, there was limited need for strict adherence to predetermined positive or negative search criteria (15). For this present study, the start of the COVID-19 pandemic was defined as November 01, 2019, a date that coincides with the initial outbreak of COVID-19 in Wuhan, China (16).

Results

A total of 114 publications were found using the search terms listed in the methods section. All articles were reviewed for relevance to the current review. 61 publications were utilized to compile this narrative review. A review of the 61 publications included in this review led to the arrangement of 6 broad categories: Definition of elective surgery; Reduction in elective surgical services during the COVID-19 Pandemic; Burden of delayed services; Ethical considerations; Moving forward; Further recommendations.

Discussion

In response to recommendations put forth by the WHO and the United States Surgeon General to halt elective procedures, healthcare providers have been faced with the challenge of protecting their patients from risks associated with COVID-19 infection by delaying elective surgical procedures. An initial challenge was simply defining exactly what constitutes an "elective" procedure. Lockey et al. (8) have discussed the arbitrary distinction between "non-elective" and "elective" surgical cases and pointed out that several so-called elective procedures are not without adverse consequences if delayed. For this discussion, the definition postulated by Commins (17) defines elective surgical procedures as those which are not immediately indicated in response to a limb- or life-threatening emergency. This definition of elective surgeries encapsulates procedures that are by no means "optional" (e.g., oncological and transplant surgeries), it simply serves to describe procedures that may be delayed without immediate threat to the life of limb.

Reduction in elective surgical services during COVID-19 pandemic

Indeed, many surgical cases were delayed on a worldwide scale in efforts to curtail the spread of COVID-19 infection. One study found admissions for elective orthopedic surgery dropped by 42% between 2019 and 2020 (18). Other authors described similar reductions in elective surgeries of 52.8% during 2020 along with a significant increase in inpatient waitlists of 73.2% for surgical procedures (19). The exact cause of reduced elective surgeries is multifaceted. Protocol changes aimed at showing the COVID-19 pandemic led to reductions in elective procedures, with stringent risk factor stratification and strict governmental policy leading to predictably increased delays (20, 21). Additional contributing factors cited for elective surgery delays include healthcare worker fatigue, relocation of staff members to COVID units, and lack of available personal protective equipment (22, 23). The positive COVID status of patients and healthcare workers was an additional contributing factor (24). Unfortunately, despite clear recommendations and the widespread availability of COVID-19 vaccines, patient compliance with preoperative vaccination has been less than optimal (25).

Burden of delayed services

Delayed patient presentation and increased time to treatment due to logistical changes which have taken place in response to the COVID-19 pandemic have led to increased burden and poorer patient outcomes (26). Delaying elective surgical procedures can lead to prolonged morbidity and exacerbation of symptoms. Some estimates suggest that more than 50% of elective surgical cases have the potential to cause significant patient harm if canceled or delayed (27). Treatment delays for elective ophthalmological procedures have raised concerns about long-term vision impairment or blindness (28). Postponed treatment of early skin lesions during the COVID-19 pandemic has led to an increased incidence of squamous cell carcinoma (29). Piketty, et al. (30) found that delays in surgical care for gynecological cancers resulted in a 9% increase in "loss of chance" (i.e., failure to treat within a timeframe that confers a reasonable likelihood of success). A meta-analysis found that postponing elective colorectal cancer cases greater than four weeks was associated with decreased overall survival and reduced disease-free survival (31). Finally, some authors argue that postponing elective surgical procedures can worsen the psychological well-being of patients who are struggling to cope with their physical health in an already strained atmosphere of fear, misinformation, and stigma (32).

It is important to consider that these surgical delays have led to a backlog of surgical waitlists that will take a considerable amount of time and labor force to ameliorate. Early estimates suggested that elective surgery waitlists would be increased by as much as 200% due to COVID-19 restraints (33). A more recent study on the subject found more conservative results of increased waitlist times of 30% above baseline upon resumption of surgical activities (9). Nonetheless, healthcare providers are concerned about the ability to manage the increased workload and costs required to reduce the backlog of patients, not to mention the increased morbidity experienced by the patients themselves (34, 35).

Ethical considerations

Healthcare providers have a moral obligation to weigh the risks versus benefits of delaying the elective surgical procedures of their patients (36). Principles of clinical ethics such as beneficence, nonmaleficence, autonomy, and justice play important roles in these considerations (8). These concepts are solidified in a survey by Campi et al. (37), which investigated varying patient perspectives on the benefits and risks of delaying surgery and underscored the importance of shared decision-making between patient and practitioner. One study found that only 56% of patients wanted to continue with previously planned elective orthopedic surgeries due to the uncertainty surrounding the COVID-19 pandemic (38), while another study by Clement et al. (39) found that the same patients who chose to defer elective procedures in the early stages of the pandemic were later amenable to surgery in the latter part of 2020 due to the lower perceived risk of contracting COVID-19. These findings highlight the importance of continued communication between patients and providers to reassess risks, benefits, and a shared understanding of treatment goals.

It has been well described that the COVID-19 pandemic has disproportionately impacted certain patient populations more than others. For example, in Louisiana, blacks make up only 32% of the population but comprise 70% of COVID-19 deaths (40). Similar trends have been observed in other areas of the United States wherein ethnic minorities surmise a disproportionate majority of COVID-19 deaths (40, 41). Considering these findings, it is important to investigate the extent to which ethnic minorities and other vulnerable sectors of society are experiencing a disproportionate burden caused by delays in elective surgical care. A study by Lin et al. (42) found that patients older than 65 years of age, non-English speakers, those with Medicare or no insurance, and those living greater than 100 miles from major healthcare facilities were disproportionately affected by the limited availability of elective surgical procedures during the COVID-19 pandemic. Another study found that racial and ethnic minorities and patients within lower-income strata are less likely to utilize telemedicine, which has occupied an increasingly larger role in healthcare delivery as the pandemic has progressed (43). A study by Bruno, Shalowitz, & Arora (44) has raised concerns over healthcare policies that aim to reduce the spread of COVID-19 but may inadvertently have negative effects on women's healthcare by assigning lower priority to elective procedures related to women's reproductive health.

Moving forward

As the COVID-19 pandemic continues to stretch, the extent to which elective surgeries should be resumed has received much attention. The COVID Surg collaborative (6), which aimed to explore the impact of COVID-19 on surgical patients and services, has suggested that surgeons consider postponing non-urgent procedures, promoting non-surgical treatments, and increasing thresholds for surgery. Other researchers have advocated for resuming elective surgical procedures. Rosati (45) proposed a structured roadmap of screening steps to guide decision-making. Many authors suggest a structured triage system to determine which patients stand to benefit most from elective surgical procedures (46, 47). The implementation of triage systems based on level stratification for elective surgeries has found success in varied clinical settings ranging from well-to-do breast clinics to resource-limited healthcare settings (48, 49). Similarly, Silva et al. (49) have proposed a risk stratification system to help guide decision-making in elective surgical cases. Importantly, performing elective surgeries after triage was not associated with increased negative short-term outcomes as evidenced by ICU admissions and mortality rates (50).

A well-structured screening procedure for detecting COVID-19 infection is an additional tool to maintain patient safety and the well-being of healthcare workers (46). Post-operative complications and increased mortality following surgery in patients infected with COVID-19 are well-documented. Patients who tested positive for COVID-19 within four weeks prior to, and up to five days after surgery exhibited increased postoperative respiratory failure, elevated scores on the Charlson Comorbidity Index, and increased mortality rates in comparison to patients who tested negative during this period (51). Up to half of the patients with perioperative COVID-19 infections experience perioperative pulmonary complications (6). There is also an increased incidence of septic shock and stroke, and overall longer hospital stays in post-operative patients infected with COVID-19 (52). This trend of increased postoperative complications and mortality has also been observed in asymptomatic patients who tested positive for COVID-19 (53). Importantly, mortality rates were similar for elective and emergency surgeries during the COVID-19 pandemic versus pre-COVID, however, patients with active COVID-19 disease exhibited mortality rates 65% greater than patients without COVID-19 disease (54). These findings suggest that it may be safe to resume elective surgical cases provided effective screening strategies are in place to avoid surgery in patients with positive COVID-19 status whenever possible. It should be noted that a limited number of studies have found no difference in mortality rates and postoperative complications in COVID-19-positive patients versus COVID-19-negative patients (55). However, considering the evidence arguing for increased postoperative complications and mortality in COVID-19-positive patients, and the potential benefits of COVID-19 screening for patients and healthcare workers, these limited studies should not be used as justification for foregoing strict COVID-19 screening procedures during the perioperative period.

Utilizing a COVID-19 screening protocol has shown positive results in securing and maintaining COVID-free surgical wards (56). Jiang and Ma (57) followed strict disinfection and screening policy to achieve zero post-operative complications or COVID-19 infections following elective, same-day surgical procedures. Screening with polymerase chain reaction (PCR) of oronasal swab samples plus chest x-ray has been mostly successful in curtailing COVID-19 infections in elective surgical candidates (58). Combination PCR testing and computed tomography (CT) imaging of the chest has been slightly more successful (59). Though, it should be cautioned that imaging alone, especially CT, should not be used as a screening tool with additional laboratory testing due to low pretest probability and substantial risk of false positive results (60). For those patients who test positive for COVID-19 during the preoperative screening period, most authors recommend delaying surgery for a minimum of four weeks for minor surgeries and up to 8-12 weeks for major surgeries (61). Additionally, post-covid patients should have recovered completely before surgery and should undergo a thorough preoperative evaluation with a special focus on parameters that assess the need for deep vein thrombosis prophylaxis and identify subclinical inflammatory states (62). One case-control study found no difference in outcomes for patients who tested positive for COVID-19 and had their surgery delayed versus those patients who tested positive for COVID-19 but did not delay surgery (63). However, based on the poorer postoperative outcomes in COVID-19-positive patients, delaying surgery should be strongly considered to protect the safety of patients and healthcare workers alike. The decision to proceed with elective surgery should be based on several factors which include, at a minimum, COVID-19 screening, analysis of comorbidities, and type of procedure (64).

Healthcare facilities that have begun moving forward with elective surgical procedures after implementing screening protocols and exercising increased preventive measures have seen positive results. One observational study of 177 patients with gastrointestinal cancer recorded zero positive cases of COVID-19 among patients and staff (65). Similarly, a case series of elective gastrointestinal procedures found no cases of COVID-19 among patients in the study and no significant increase in postoperative complications compared to pre-pandemic rates (66).

Further recommendations

The COVID-19 pandemic has spurred a rapid surge in the utilization of distance care and telemedicine (2, 3). Authors have advocated for the use of telemedicine in the realm of elective surgeries both in the pre-and postoperative periods (67, 68). Telemedicine is not without certain drawbacks. It requires secure teleconferencing software and additional legal and risk-management considerations to ensure patient safety and confidentiality (69). Additionally, as mentioned above, there still exists disparities in access to and/or willingness to engage in telemedicine (43). Despite any potential shortcomings, telemedicine has been well-received during the COVID-19 pandemic. A recent meta-analysis found no differences between telemedicine and in-person appointments for in-patient satisfaction scores, surgeon satisfaction scores, and patient-reported outcome measures; however, note that this study did not address objective safety endpoints (70).

In addition to telemedicine, authors suggest the use of outpatient and same-day surgery centers to avoid spreading COVID-19 infection (71, 72). One study showed promising results by incorporating elective surgical care into a “hub-and-spoke” model wherein local and regional hub centers could provide surgical care in settings that have minimal COVID-19 burden in comparison to hospitals and inpatient settings (73). Moving forward, considerations for elective surgeries should include a focus on resource availability, patient fitness, and time sensitivity of procedures while utilizing telemedicine and outpatient facilities when possible (74).

Conclusion

The COVID-19 pandemic has led to a significant shift in the delivery of elective surgical care (18, 19). Delays in the timely delivery of elective surgeries along with complications caused by SARS-CoV-2 infection have led to poorer patient outcomes and an increased burden on healthcare workers (22, 23, 26). As elective surgeries are resumed and the backlog of surgical waitlists is addressed, surgeons must weigh the ethical and safety considerations of proceeding with elective surgeries. Strong screening protocols for COVID-19 disease along with the utilization of outpatient surgical centers and telemedicine offer a pathway for moving forward (56, 67).

References

[1] Moynihan R, Sanders S, Michaleff ZA, Scott AM, Clark J, To EJ, et al. Impact of COVID-19 pandemic on utilization of healthcare services: a systematic review. BMJ Open 2021;11(3):e045343.

[2] Bate NJ, Xu SC, Pacilli M, Roberts LJ, Kimber C, Nataraja RM. Effect of the COVID-19-induced phase of massive telehealth uptake on end-user satisfaction. Intern Med J 2021;51(2):206-14.

[3] Koonin LM, Hoots B, Tsang CA, Leroy Z, Farris K, Jolly T, et al. Trends in the use of telehealth during the emergence of the COVID-19 pandemic - United States, January-March 2020. MMWR 2020;69(43):1595-9.

[4] De Simone B, Chouillard E, Di Saverio S, Pagani L, Sartelli M, Biffl WL, et al. Emergency surgery during the COVID-19 pandemic: What you need to know for practice. Ann R Coll Surg Engl 2020;102(5):323-32.

[5] Hu S, Wang W, Wang Y, Litvinova M, Luo K, Ren L, et al. Infectivity, susceptibility, and risk factors associated with SARS-CoV-2 transmission under intensive contact tracing in Hunan, China. Nat Commun 2021;12(1):2251.

[6] COVIDSurg Collaborative. Mortality and pulmonary complications in patients undergoing surgery with perioperative SARS-CoV-2 infection: an international cohort study. Lancet 2020;396(10243):27-38.

[7] World Health Organization. COVID-19: Operational guidance for maintaining essential health services during an outbreak: interim guidance. Geneva: World Health Organization, 2020.

[8] Lockey SD, Nelson PC, Kessler MJ, & Kessler MW. Approaching "elective" Surgery in the Era of COVID-19. J Hand Surg Am 2020;46(1):60–4.

[9] Uimonen M, Kuitunen I, Paloneva J, Launonen AP, Ponkilainen V, Mattila VM. The impact of the COVID-19 pandemic on waiting times for elective surgery patients: A multicenter study. PLoS One 2021;16(7): e0253875.

[10] Metelmann IB, Busemann A. Elective surgery in times of COVID-19: A two-center analysis of postponed operations and disease-related morbidity and mortality. Z Evid Fortbild Qual Gesundhwes 2020;158-159:62-5.

[11] Byrnes ME, Brown CS, De Roo AC, Corriere MA, Romano MA, Fukuhara S, et al. Elective surgical delays due to COVID-19: The patient lived experience. Med Care 2021;59(4):288-94.

[12] Forner D, Murnaghan S, Porter G, Mason RJ, Hong P, Taylor SM, et al. Psychosocial distress in adult patients awaiting cancer surgery during the COVID-19 pandemic. Curr Oncol 2021;28(3):1867-78.

[13] Oudhoff JP, Timmermans DR, Knol DL, Bijnen AB, van der Wal G. Waiting for elective general surgery: impact on health-related quality of life and psychosocial consequences. BMC Public Health 2007;7:164.

[14] Johnson CL, Schwartz H, Greenberg A, Hernandez S, Nnamani Silva ON, Wong LE, et al. Patient Perceptions on Barriers and Facilitators to Accessing Low-acuity Surgery During COVID-19 Pandemic. J Surg Res 2021;264:30-6.

[15] Grant MJ, Booth A. A typology of reviews: An analysis of 14 review types and associated methodologies. Health Info Libr J 2009;26(2):91-108.

[16] Sun J, He WT, Wang L, Lai A, Ji X, Zhai X, etbal. COVID-19: Epidemiology, evolution, and cross-disciplinary perspectives. Trends Mol Med 2020;26(5):483-95.

[17] Commins J. Surgeon general urges providers to ‘consider sStopping all eElective surgeries.’ Hospitals push back. Health Leaders 2020 Mar 16. URL: https://www.healthleadersmedia.com/clinical-care/surgeon-general-urges-providers-consider-stopping-elective-surgeries-hospitals-push.

[18] Zagra L, Faraldi M, Andreata M, Ottaiano I, Basile G, Lombardi G. A seven-week observational analysis of clinical activities in a North Italian orthopedic hospital during the second wave of SARS-CoV-2 pandemic: far from usual volumes, but different from the first wave. Int Orthop 2021;45(10):2473-82.

[19] Hampton M, Riley E, Garneti N, Anderson A, Wembridge K. The orthopedic waiting list crisis: Two sides of the story. Bone Jt Open 2021;2(7):530-4.

[20] Truche P, Campos LN, Marrazzo EB, Rangel AG, Bernardino R, Bowder AN, et al. Association between government policy and delays in emergent and elective surgical care during the COVID-19 pandemic in Brazil: a modeling study. Lancet Reg Health Am 2021;3:100056.

[21] Din N, Phylactou M, Fajardo-Sanchez J, Watson M, Ahmad S. The impact of COVID-19 on acute and elective corneal surgery at Moorfields Eye Hospital London. Clin Ophthalmol 2021;15:1639-45.

[22] Santoro GA, Grossi U, Murad-Regadas S, Nunoo-Mensah JW, Mellgren A, Di Tanna vG L, et al. Delayed colorectal cancer care during COVID-19 pandemic (DECOR-19): Global perspective from an international survey. Surgery 2020;169(4):796–807.

[23] Whelehan DF, Connelly TM, Ridgway PF. COVID-19 and surgery: A thematic analysis of unintended consequences on performance, practice, and surgical training. Surgeon 2021;19(1): e20-7.

[24] Søreide K, Hallet J, Matthews JB, Schnitzbauer AA, Line PD, Lai P, et al. Immediate and long-term impact of the COVID-19 pandemic on delivery of surgical services. Br J Surg 2020;107(10):1250–61.

[25] Anwar SL, Cahyono R, Hardiyanto H, Suwardjo S, Darwito D, Harahap WA. The prioritation and gap of preoperative COVID-19 vaccination in cancer surgery of the breast, head and neck, and skin: A cohort study of 367 patients in an Indonesian hospital. Ann Med Surg (Lond) 2021;72:103089.

[26] Khan R, Zaidi N, Chituku T, Rao M. Non-COVID fatalities in the COVID era: A paradigm shift in the face of a pandemic-lessons learnt (or not). Ann Med Surg (Lond) 2021;70:102617.

[27] Zhang S. What it really means to cancel elective surgeries. Atlantic 2020 Mar 17. URL: https://www.theatlantic.com/science/archive/2020/03/patients-whose-surgeries-are-canceled-because-coronavirus/608176/.

[28] Toro MD, Brézin AP, Burdon M, Cummings AB, Evren Kemer O, Malyugin BE, et al. Early impact of COVID-19 outbreaks on eye care: Insights from EUROCOVCAT group. Eur J Ophthalmol 2021;31(1):5-9.

[29] Seretis K, Boptsi E, Boptsi A, Lykoudis EG. The impact of treatment delay on skin cancer in COVID-19 era: a case-control study. World J Surg Oncol 2021;19(1):350.

[30] Piketty J, Carbonnel M, Murtada R, Revaux A, Asmar J, Favre-Inhofer A, et al. Collateral damage of COVID-19 pandemic: The impact on a gynecologic surgery department. J Gynecol Obstet Hum Reprod 2022;51(1):102255.

[31] Whittaker TM, Abdelrazek MEG, Fitzpatrick AJ, Froud JLJ, Kelly JR, Williamson JS, Williams GL. Delay to elective colorectal cancer surgery and implications for survival: a systematic review and meta-analysis. Colorectal Dis 2021;23(7):1699-711.

[32] Ren SY, Gao RD, Chen YL. Fear can be more harmful than the severe acute respiratory syndrome coronavirus 2 in controlling the corona virus disease 2019 epidemic. World J Clin Cases 2020;8(4):652-7.

[33] Salenger R, Etchill EW, Ad N, Matthew T, Alejo D, Whitman G, et al. The surge after the surge: Cardiac surgery post-COVID-19. Ann Thorac Surg 2020;110(6):2020-5.

[34] Fowler AJ, Dobbs TD, Wan YI, Laloo R, Hui S, Nepogodiev D, et al. Resource requirements for reintroducing elective surgery during the COVID-19 pandemic: modelling study. Br J Surg 2021;108(1):97-103.

[35] Rubicon F, Cohen RV, Mingrone G, le Roux CW, Mechanick JI, Arterburn DE, et al. Bariatric and metabolic surgery during and after the COVID-19 pandemic: DSS recommendations for management of surgical candidates and postoperative patients and prioritisation of access to surgery. Lancet Diabetes Endocrinol 2020;8(7):640–8.

[36] Macleod J, Mezher S, Hasan R. Surgery during COVID-19 crisis conditions: Can we protect our ethical integrity against the odds? J Med Ethics 2020;46(8):505-7.

[37] Campi R, Tellini R, Grosso AA, Amparore D, Mari A, Viola L, et al. Deferring elective urologic surgery during the COVID-19 pandemic: The patients' perspective. Urology 2021;147:21-6.

[38] Chang J, Wignadasan W, Kontoghiorghe C, Kayani B, Singh S, Plastow R, et al. Restarting elective orthopaedic services during the COVID-19 pandemic: Do patients want to have surgery? Bone Jt Open 2020;1(6):267-71.

[39] Clement ND, Oussedik S, Raza KI, Patton RFL, Smith K, Deehan DJ. The rate of patient deferral and barriers to going forward with elective orthopaedic surgery during the COVID-19 pandemic. Bone Jt Open 2020;1(10):663-8.

[40] Artiga S, Garfield R, Orgera K. Communities of color at higher risk for health and economic challenges due to COVID-19. United States: KFF, 2020. URL: https://www.kff.org/coronavirus-covid-19/issue-brief/communities-of-color-at-higher-risk-for-health-and-economic-challenges-due-to-covid-19/.

[41] Godoy M, Wood D. What do coronavirus racial disparities look like state by state? Npr 2020 May 30. URL: https://www.npr.org/sections/health-shots/2020/05/30/865413079/what-do-coronavirus-racial-disparities-look-like-state-by-state.

[42] Lin JA, Braun HJ, Schwab ME, Pierce L, Sosa JA, Wick EC. Pandemic recovery: Persistent disparities in access to elective surgical procedures. Ann Surg 2021;10.1097/SLA.0000000000004848.

[43] Whaley CM, Pera MF, Cantor J, Chang J, Velasco J, Hagg HK, et al. Changes in health services use among commercially insured US populations during the COVID-19 pandemic. JAMA Netw Open 2020;3(11): e2024984.

[44] Bruno B, Shalowitz DI, Arora KS. Ethical challenges for women's healthcare highlighted by the COVID-19 pandemic. J Med Ethics 2021;47(2):69-72.

[45] Rosati F, Muneretto C, Baudo M, D'Ancona G, Bichi S, Merlo M, et al. A multicentre roadmap to restart elective cardiac surgery after COVID-19 peak in an Italian epicenter. J Card Surg 2021;36(9):3308–16.

[46] Gok AFK, Eryılmaz M, Ozmen MM, Alimoglu O, Ertekin C, Kurtoglu MH. Recommendations for trauma and emergency general surgery practice during COVID-19 pandemic. Ulus Travma Acil Cerrahi Derg 2020;26(3):335-42.

[47] Alipour S, Moini A, Orouji M, Saberi A, Motamedi M, Eskandari A. COVID-19 outbreak and consequent delays in schedules of the Breast Clinic: Effects on patients' breast and emotional symptoms. Eur J Breast Health 2020;16(4):25054.

[48] Windon MJ, Faniriko MBA, Bogale M, Acha E, Koch W. Otolaryngology burden of disease and surgical case triage in resource-limited settings: An example from Cameroon. Laryngoscope Investig Otolaryngol 2021;6(2):177-82.

[49] Silva LED, Cohen RV, DE-Andrade JC, SzegÖ T, Santo MA, Ramos AC, etbal The recommendations of the Brazilian College of Surgeons and the Brazilian Bariatric and Metabolic Surgery Societies on the return of bariatric and metabolic operations in geographic regions of the country where the procedures have been allowed by local policies, in the period of COVID-19 pandemic. Rev Col Bras Cir 2020;47 e20202640.

[50] Durand M, Bentellis I, Barthe F, Tibi B, Shaikh A, Mellouki A, etbal. Évaluation des mesures de triages de la première vague pandémique Covid-19 pour sélectionner les patients à opérer pour cancers et urgences urologiques [Outcomes following the triage of patients for urological cancer and non-cancer surgery during Covid-19 pandemic peak]. Prog Urol 2021;31(12):716-24. [French]

[51] Kiyatkin ME, Levine SP, Kimura A, Linzer RW, Labins JR, Kim JI, et bal. Increased incidence of post-operative respiratory failure in patients with pre-operative SARS-CoV-2 infection. J Clin Anesth 2021; 74:110409.

[52] Lal BK, Prasad NK, Englum BR, Turner DJ, Siddiqui T, Carlin MM, etbal. Periprocedural complications in patients with SARS-CoV-2 infection compared to those without infection: A nationwide propensity-matched analysis. Am J Surg 2021;222(2):431-7.

[53] Patkar S, Voppuru SR, Thiagarajan S, Niyogi D, Niranjan HS, Nadkarni S, etbal. Incidence of SARS-CoV-2 infection among asymptomatic patients undergoing preoperative COVID testing prior to cancer surgery: ASPECT study. J Surg Oncol 2022;125(4):564-9.

[54] Tavanaei R, Ahmadi P, Yazdani KO, Zali A, Oraee-Yazdani S. The impact of the coronavirus disease 2019 pandemic on neurosurgical practice and feasibility of safe resumption of elective procedures during this era in a large referral center in Tehran, Iran: An unmatched case-control study. World Neurosurg 2021;154: e370-81.

[55] Vosburg RW, Pratt JSA, Kindel T, Rogers AM, Kudav S, Banerjee A, et al. Bariatric surgery is safe for patients after recovery from COVID-19. Surg Obes Relat Dis 2021;17(11):1884-9.

[56] Brar S, Ofo E, Hyde N, Kim D, Odutoye T, Allin D, etbal. Outcomes of elective head and neck confirmed or suspected cancer surgery during the COVID-19 pandemic. Eur Arch Otorhinolaryngol 2021;278(4):1277-82.

[57] Jiang L, Ma H. Surgical protocol in a West China Day Surgery Center during the COVID-19 pandemic: Practice and experience. Surg Innov 2020;28(1):53–7.

[58] Kane AD, Paterson J, Pokhrel S, Berry SK, Monkhouse D, Brand JW, etbal. Peri-operative COVID-19 infection in urgent elective surgery during a pandemic surge period: a retrospective observational cohort study. Anaesthesia 2020;75(12):1596-604.

[59] Guerlain J, Haroun F, Voicu A, Honoré C, Griscelli F, Temam S, et al. Cancer surgery during the COVID-19 pandemic: The experience of a comprehensive cancer center performing preoperative screening by RT-PCR and chest CT scan. J Surg Oncol 2021;123(4):815–22.

[60] Ap Dafydd D, O'Mahony M, Jhanji S, Devaraj A, Allum W, Nicol D, et al. The role of CT chest in screening for asymptomatic COVID-19 infection in self-isolating patients prior to elective oncological surgery: findings from a UK Cancer Hub. Br J Radiol 2021;94(1117):20200994.

[61] Kovoor JG, Scott NA, Tivey DR, Babidge WJ, Scott DA, Beavis VS, et al. Proposed delay for safe surgery after COVID-19. Aust NZ J Surg 2021;91(4):495-506.

[62] Tunescu M, Christodorescu R, Sharma A, Barsac CR, Rogobete AF, Crisan DC, et al. The preoperative evaluation of post-COVID-19 patients scheduled for elective surgery - What is important not to miss! Eur Rev Med Pharmacol Sci 2021;25(23):7607-15.

[63] Baiocchi G, Aguiar S Jr, Duprat JP, Coimbra F, Makdissi FB, Vartanian JG, et al. Early postoperative outcomes among patients with delayed surgeries after a preoperative positive test for SARS-CoV-2: A case-control study from a single institution. J Surg Oncol 2020;123(4):823–33.

[64] Attia AK, Omar UF, Kaliya-Perumal AK. A review of guidelines to resuming elective orthopaedic surgeries amid COVID-19 pandemic: Deriving a simple traffic light model. Malays Orthop J 2020;14(3):10-5.

[65] Sozutek A, Seker A, Kuvvetli A, Ozer N, Genc IC. Evaluating the feasibility of performing elective gastrointestinal cancer surgery during the COVID-19 pandemic: An observational study with 60 days follow-up results of a tertiary referral pandemic hospital. J Surg Oncol 2021;123(4):834-41.

[66] Kapoor D, Perwaiz A, Singh A, Chaudhary A. Elective gastrointestinal surgery in COVID times. Indian J Surg 2021;83(1):277-83.

[67] Bonillo-García MÁ, Morán-Pascual E, Puche-Sanz I, Campos-Juanatey F, Martínez-Piñeiro L, Ponce de León-Roca J. Recomendaciones de actuación en cirugía reconstructiva urológica durante la pandemia Covid-19 [Reconstructive surgery protocol recommendations during COVID-19 pandemia.]. Arch Esp Urol 2020;73(5):413-9. [Spanish]

[68] Tasa D, Eslami P, Dashti H, Nassiri Toosi M, Zarghami SY, Zarghami SY, et al. The successful management of Thirty-six hepatopancreatobiliary surgeries under the intensive protective arrangements during the COVID-19 pandemic. Acta Biomed 2020;91(3):e2020005.

[69] De Santis G, Palladino T, Leti Acciaro A, Starnoni M. The telematic solutions in plastic surgery during the COVID-19 pandemic. Acta Biomed 2020;91(3): e2020053.

[70] Chaudhry H, Nadeem S, Mundi R. How satisfied are patients and Surgeons with telemedicine in orthopaedic care during the COVID-19 pandemic? A systematic review and meta-analysis. Clin Orthop Relat Res 2021;479(1):47–56.

[71] Ding BTK, Decruz J, Kunnasegaran R. Time-sensitive ambulatory orthopaedic soft-tissue surgery paradigms during the COVID-19 pandemic. Int Orthop 2020;44(8):1531-8.

[72] Shao CC, McLeod MC, Gleason L, Marques ICDS, Chu DI, Gunnells D. Effect of COVID-19 pandemic restructuring on surgical volume and outcomes of non-COVID patients undergoing surgery. Am Surg 2022;88(3):489-97.

[73] Kasivisvanathan R, Tilney HS, Jhanji S, O'Mahony M, Gruber P, Nicol D, et al. The 'hub and spoke model' for the management of surgical patients during the COVID-19 pandemic. Int J Health Plann Manage 2021;36(5):1397–406.

[74] Comfort SM, Murata Y, Pierpoint LA, Philippon MJ. Management of outpatient elective surgery for arthroplasty and sports medicine during the COVID-19 pandemic: A scoping review. Orthop J Sports Med 2021;9(11): 23259671211 053335.

Chapter 12

Dengue vaccine development and safety: What went wrong?

Barry A Eagel, MD, MPH
Anthony La, BA
Deepak Kumar Palanichami, BSc
Gerard St Cyr, MPH, MSc
Lauren Orlando, PhD
Abidemi Fasanmi, MD, MPH, PhD
and Emmanuel O Keku*, MD, MA, MSPH
School of Medicine, Department of Public Health and Preventive Medicine, St George's University, St George, Grenada, West Indies

Abstract

Dengue infection is caused by the bite of an infected mosquito carrying one of four dengue virus variants. In 2015, the first vaccine for dengue fever, Dengvaxia® (Sanofi-Pasteur) was approved. Its indication was limited to prior dengue fever infections to prevent severe dengue, due to serious adverse effects seen during the Phase 3 trials with dengue seronegative subjects. The reasons for those serious adverse events were evaluated by a focused literature review. Literature searches of five databases identified clinical studies and reviews that were relevant to the drug approval, safety, and efficacy of dengue vaccines, and found a total of 830 articles, of which there were 25 clinical trials of dengue vaccines. Review of the clinical trials and subsequent safety analyses showed that

* Corresponding Author's Email: ekeku@sgu.edu.

In: Public Health
Editors: Emmanuel O Keku and Joav Merrick
ISBN: 979-8-89113-083-8

either transmission of dengue virus through a mosquito bite or immunization may create partial immunity to some dengue subtypes, and non-neutralizing antibodies formed may facilitate viral replication, increasing the likelihood of severe dengue sequelae. The limits of the current approved vaccine and alternatives will be reviewed. Increased morbidity and mortality were due to antibody-dependent enhancement caused by the vaccine. Individual testing for dengue antibodies before vaccination is safer than reliance on population seroprevalence rates.

Keywords: dengue, dengue fever, dengue vaccine, antibody-dependent enhancement, epidemiology, clinical trial, pharmacovigilance, post-marketing safety surveillance

Introduction

Dengue is an acute syndrome characterized by fever, headache, myalgias and rash caused by one of four variants of a flavivirus, (DENV-1, - 2, -3 and -4) transmitted by the bite of a female *Aedes* species mosquito (1). The incubation and viremic period after the bite of the female *Aedes ægypti* mosquito and transfer of the dengue virus into the blood, is three to 14 days, during which the patient is viremic and infectious. Only 20% of infections present with symptoms of fever, joint and muscle pain, skin rash, nausea, and headache (1, 2).

Infection with one of the four strains can confer immunity to that strain, but only partial immunity to the other three strains, which wanes over two to three years (3), and re-infection with one of the other strains can cause a more severe form of dengue: dengue hemorrhagic fever (DHF) or dengue shock syndrome (DSS), characterized by increased vascular permeability, hypovolemic shock, disseminated intravascular coagulation, and thrombocytopenia (4).

Dengue is estimated to afflict one million persons per day, is a reportable illness and is considered by the WHO as a public health concern (5, 6). With no effective curative treatment except supportive care, several vaccine candidates have been developed against all four dengue variant subtypes. In 2015, one vaccine was approved by the World Health Organization (WHO). A mass vaccination program in the Philippines resulted in excess hospitalizations and deaths in school aged children (7).

Epidemiology of dengue

The potential endemic global area encompasses nearly four billion people (8, 9), causing up to 390 million infections annually (10), 100 million cases of symptomatic dengue infection, with an annual mortality rate of 40,000 people (8). Over the past 50 years, the global incidence of dengue has increased by 30-fold (11). It is most seen in tropical and subtropical areas, however, global risks of dengue virus spreading to non-endemic areas have increased due to global warming, globalization, and urbanization (1, 2). It is the most common mosquito transmitted arbovirus in the world, affecting 128 countries (10), and will increase the worldwide population at risk of dengue to 6.1 billion people, or 60% of the global population in the next 60 years (12).

Molecular biology of the dengue virus

Dengue is a flavivirus in the same genus as yellow fever, West Nile fever, and Zika viruses. Dengue is a single strand of positive-sense RNA, which codes for 10 viral proteins: the envelope protein (E), the capsid (C), the membrane (coded as the pre-membrane protein prM), and 7 non-structural proteins (NS). The glycoprotein capsule is composed of the membrane and the envelope (E) proteins (3), see Figure 1.

The dengue virus has four distinct serotypes which affect humans, referred to as DENV-1, DENV-2, DENV-3 and DENV-4. The virus is transmitted by the bite of the female *Aedes ægypti* mosquito, although the *Aedes albopictus* mosquito is also a vector in some areas of the world. A fifth serotype, DENV-5 was reported in 2013 in a Malaysian patient (12, 13) however it is believed this variant only has a non-human sylvatic life cycle (1, 14). The virus is transmitted to the mosquito after biting an infected host while viremic, which can occur up to two days before symptoms of fever begin. The virus then travels to the salivary glands of the female *Aedes* mosquito where it can infect another person with the same serotype variant of dengue. Following recovery, serotype specific memory T and B cells are formed, which produce neutralizing antibodies to the specific serotype variant that caused the infection, with limited cross-reactivity to the other three serotypes which wanes over two to three years.

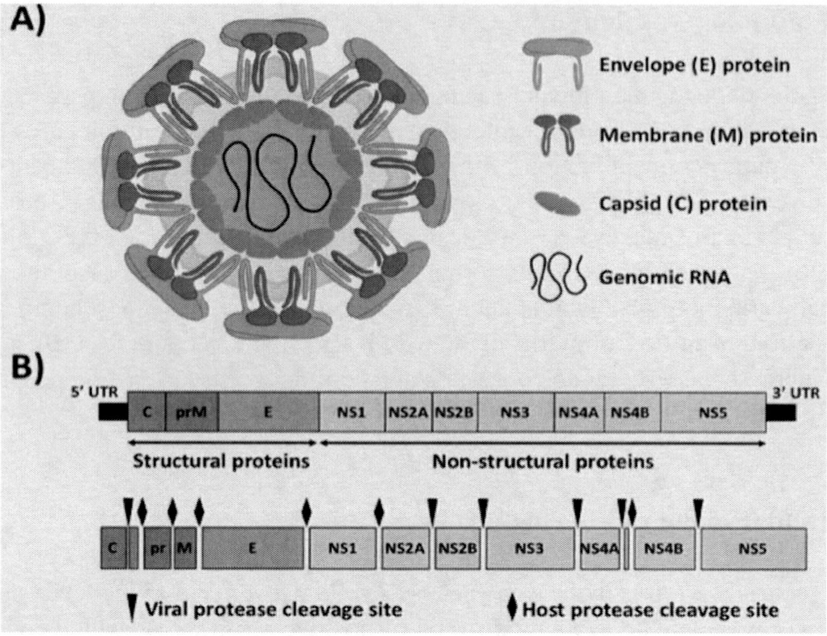

Figure 1. (A) Flavivirus structure showing envelope protein, capsid protein, and RNA strand. (B) Schematic of RNA genome divided into ten open reading frames (ORF) regions. NS= non-structural ORF domains.

Immunologic responses

Initial infection with any one of the four DENV serotypes causes a self-limited febrile illness, dengue fever, which resolves within several days. This viral infection causes production of neutralizing IgM and then IgG antibodies to the specific serotype (see Figure 2), and confers immunity to the same serotype, but only partial and limited immunity to subsequent infection with other serotypes in the same patient (15). This is due to non-specific binding of the antibodies to the other serotypes, which can enhance the entry of the virus into innate immune cells (monocytes and macrophages) during the subsequent infection (16). This results in a higher viremic load, vascular leakage, and thrombocytopenia, leading to more severe forms of dengue, dengue hemorrhagic fever or dengue shock syndrome, depending on whether the destruction of platelets (thrombocytopenia) or vascular leakage (hypovolemic shock) predominates. The enhanced viral infectivity due to non-neutralizing antibodies is termed *antibody-dependent enhancement* (ADE) (see Figure 3) (3, 16-18).

Second infection with a different serotype strain may cause severe dengue, due to the presence of non-neutralizing antibodies from the original infectious strain (see Figure 3 C, D). These non-neutralizing antibodies promote enhanced viral entry into monocytes and macrophages, where the virus replicates and increases the viremic load. Release of cytokines due to T cell activation promotes capillary leakage, leading to hypovolemia seen in dengue shock syndrome, and hemostatic abnormalities including thrombocytopenia and petechiae characteristic of dengue hemorrhagic fever (1, 19, 20).

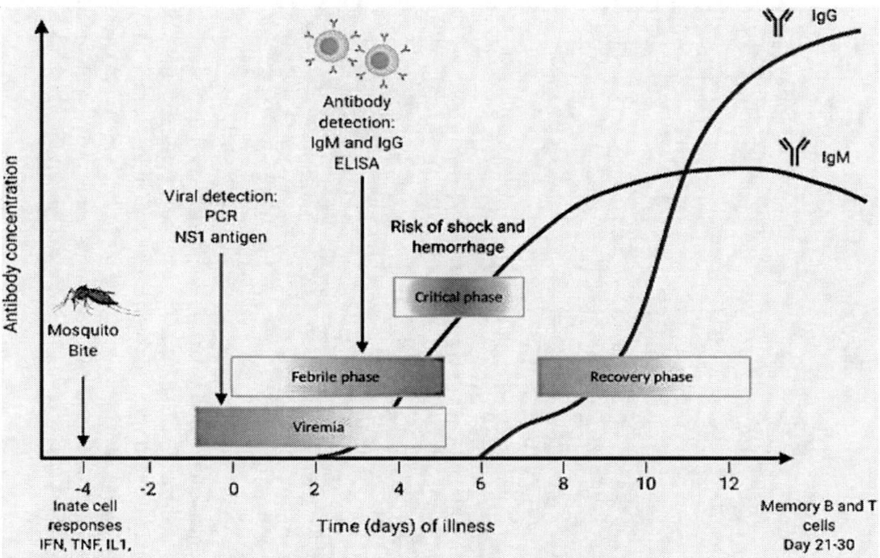

Source: https://www.frontiersin.org/files/Articles/542949/fimmu-11-01055-HTML/image_m/fimmu-11-01055-g001.jpg.

Figure 2. Time course of infection with dengue, immunologic responses, and clinical course.

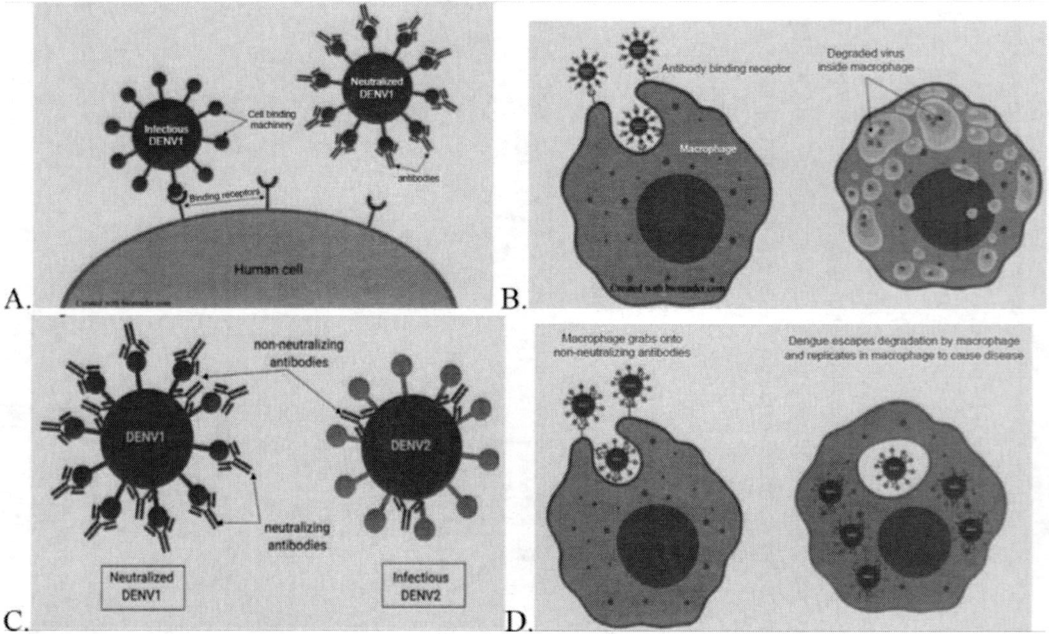

Source: BioRender.com.

Figure 3. Antibody dependent enhancement (ADE). A. In response to an infection with DENV-1 virus, B-cells make serotype specific anti-DENV-1 neutralizing antibodies, which attach on human macrophage cells. B. DENV coated with neutralizing antibodies is phagocytized by macrophages. C. During a second infection with a different serotype, in this case, DENV-2, memory B cells make anti-DENV-1 antibodies with only partial cross- reactivity with DENV-2 viruses. D. These partially cross-reactive antibodies are non-neutralizing. They promote phagocytosis by macrophages but not destruction of the virus. When the virus coated with non-neutralizing antibodies enters the macrophage, the viral RNA incorporates into the nucleic acid material of the cell, manufacturing more copies of the viral proteins, enhancing the production of new viruses.

Problem statement

The cause of the cases of severe dengue and death attributed to the approved Dengvaxia vaccine resulted from vaccination of seronegative people, some who may have been false positive by self-reporting, which may be due to antibody-dependent enhancement resulting from viral interference and unequal dengue serotype antibody production.

Research question

Does the currently approved dengue vaccine cause excess morbidity and mortality in some people, why does this occur and how can it be prevented? This focused, narrative literature reviewed published articles on the development of dengue vaccines, discusses the reasons for vaccine-related adverse events and reviews the status of ongoing research to develop a safer, more effective dengue vaccine.

Methods

Literature searches were conducted using Medline via PubMed, ScienceDirect, Cochrane Database of Systematic Reviews, Google Scholar and Web of Science for clinical trials or systematic reviews for drug safety related to dengue vaccines.

Inclusion criteria

1. (Drug approval, drug safety, pharmacovigilance, or adverse events) AND (dengue vaccines, dengue fever, severe dengue, dengue haemorrhagic fever or dengue shock syndrome)
2. Limited to humans, English language, full text and published within the last 10 years
3. Clinical trials or systematic reviews with meta-analyses

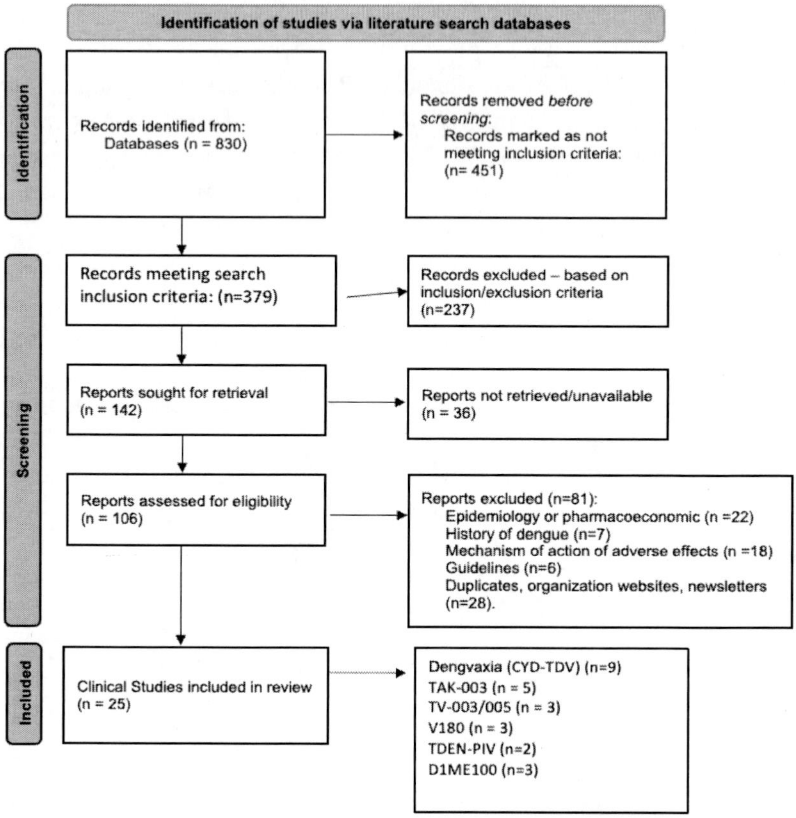

Figure 4. PRISMA flow diagram for dengue vaccine search criteria and results. Modified from: Page MJ, McKenzie JE, Bossuyt PM, Boutron I, Hoffmann TC, Mulrow CD, et al. (21). The PRISMA 2020 statement: An updated guideline for reporting systematic reviews. BMJ 2021;372: n71. doi: 10.1136/bmj. n71 https://www.prisma-statement.org/PRISMAStatement/FlowDiagram.aspx.

Exclusion criteria

Unpublished results from websites, review articles without statistical analysis, editorials, guidelines, letters, trials of combination vaccinations (e.g., with influenza or MMR vaccines). The Boolean search criteria used for PubMed was: ("dengue"[MeSH Major Topic]) OR ("dengue virus"[MeSH Major Topic])) OR ("dengue fever"[All Fields] OR "dengue fever dengue hemorrhagic fever"[All Fields])) OR (dengue)) AND ((("dengue vaccines" [MeSH Major Topic]) OR ("dengue vaccines/ pharmacology" [MeSH Major

Topic])) OR ("dengue vaccines/adverse effects"[MeSH Major Topic])) AND (("clinical trial"[ALL FIELDS]) or ("clinical trial" [MeSH]))

- N = 830
- Limited to full English text, last 10 years = 379
- Limited to clinical trials OR meta-analysis OR randomized controlled trial or systemic review, limited to past 10 years, full English text, N = 142,
- Available in library and non-duplicated, N = 106

Additional research was done for epidemiology, pharmacoeconomic, history of dengue fever, and mechanisms of action for serious adverse effects during the clinical trials. In addition, an independent search was conducted of the St George's University Founders Library holdings for graduate theses focused on dengue in Grenada. This search yielded a further four master's degree theses and one doctoral thesis manuscript, see Figure 4.

Results

- Twenty-five articles discussed dengue clinical trials (see Figure 1 and Table 1).
  - Nine articles discussed the Sanofi-Pasteur Dengvaxia® CYD-TDV vaccine clinical trials:
    - Four papers presented results of multiple trials: Lang (22) reviewed the phase 1 trials, Thomas and Yoon (23) presented the results of 26 Phase 1, 2 and 3 trials, Guy (24) presented the results of a Phase 2b, and two Phase 3 studies, and Tully and Griffiths presented the results of 7 Phase 2 and 3 trials (25):
  - There was one Phase 1 PK/PD study (26), a Phase 2 (27), 2b RCT (28), two Phase 3 RCTs (29, 30), and a single retrospective cohort trial (26).
- Six articles discussed dengue trial guidelines in general (3, 6, 31-35).
- Twenty-two articles dealt with epidemiology or pharmacoeconomic factors related to dengue and were used for background information.
- Seven articles related to the history of dengue fever epidemics and pandemics.

- Eighteen articles contained discussions about the mechanism of action and causes of the cases of severe dengue seen during the clinical trials and the etiology of vaccine antibody dependent enhancement.
- Ponndorf reviewed pharmacokinetic data from a novel tobacco leaf virus-like protein which mimicked nonspecific (NS) proteins of the DENV (36).
- The remaining papers provided information on mosquito control, management of severe dengue, or were non-peer reviewed articles (e.g., news articles, editorials, websites, etc.).
- The search of the Founders Library for thesis manuscripts from graduate students at St. George's University focused on dengue in Grenada yielded four Master of Science degrees (20, 37-40) and one Doctoral thesis (41) manuscripts.

There were no safety concerns noted during the Phase 1 or 2 trials of Dengvaxia. In the two Phase 3 studies, the incidence of systemic adverse events in the vaccine groups was 67%, compared to 59% in the placebo group (42, 43).

Among seropositive vaccines, the number of cases of hospitalization decreased by 15 per 1,000, while the incidence of severe Dengue decreased by 5 per 1,000 (57). However, in the seronegative group, a 5-year follow-up showed that about five additional hospitalized dengue cases or two additional severe Dengue cases per 1,000 vaccinees in seronegatives could occur following vaccination compared to unvaccinated seronegative children (58, 59). The relative risk for hospitalization or severe dengue in the seropositive group was 0.18 (95% CI [0.09, 0.37]), compared to 6.25 [0.81, 48.32] in seronegative subjects (60). Hospitalization in seronegative people could either be due to ineffectiveness of the vaccine in preventing dengue, since the vaccine efficacy during the clinical trials was only ~60%, or due to a vaccine-associated enhanced viral syndrome, known as *antibody-dependent enhancement* (ADE), described in detail *supra vide* and in Figure 3. During the clinical trials, the hospitalizations in seronegative vaccines were attributed to breakthrough infection only, and only after analysis of safety data post-market approval, was the alternative ADE adverse event considered. Flasche et al. (41) estimated that by 5 years after vaccination in the Philippines cohort of school age vaccines, 52% of hospitalizations would occur in children seropositive before vaccination who had breakthrough dengue secondary infections, due to low vaccine efficacy. Of the 42% of seronegative people who were vaccinated who were hospitalized, one-third would have had vaccine-associated ADE and two-thirds would have been due to breakthrough infections. They also stated that for every case of dengue hospitalization caused by the vaccine in seronegative, 18 cases of dengue hospitalization would be prevented in seropositive vaccines, and for every case of severe dengue in seronegative caused by the vaccine, 10 cases of severe dengue would be prevented in seropositive.

Discussion

Since 1945, attempts have been made to develop a vaccine for dengue (15, 61). In 2006, clinical trials were started on a chimeric recombinant live attenuated tetravalent dengue vaccine by Sanofi-Pasteur, CYD-TDV (Dengvaxia®). The backbone of the CYD vaccine was the live attenuated 17D-YF strain which had been used for yellow fever vaccines since 1937 (62). The 17D yellow fever strain provided the 7 non-structural (NS) and the C coding regions of the CYD-TDV dengue vaccine, while the pre-membrane (prM) and E proteins from each of the four DENV serotypes was substituted for the prM and E regions on the yellow fever RNA (see Figure 5).

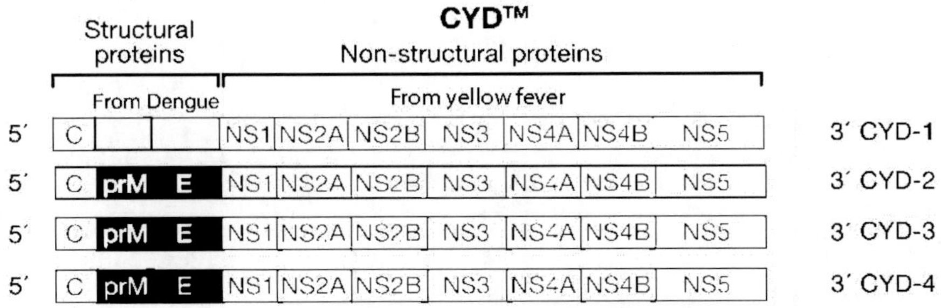

Figure 5. Genome structure of CYD-TDV (Dengvaxia®) live attenuated chimeric tetravalent dengue vaccine (61). C = capsid; prM = pre-Membrane; E = envelope protein; NS1, -2A, -2B, -3, -4A, -4B, -5 = non-structural protein; CYD = chimeric yellow fever-dengue; CYD-1, -2, -3, -4 = chimeric yellow fever 17D strain virus RNA backbone, with dengue DENV-1, -2, -3, -4 prM and E ORF regions spliced into YF RNA.

Table 1. Dengue vaccine candidates in clinical trials

Vaccine Type	Vaccine Name	Developer	Current Stage	Strategy	Key Clinical Outcome	Ref
Live attenuated	Dengvaxia® (CYD-TDV)	Sanofi-Pasteur	Licensed	DENV 1–4 prM/E genes substituted on YF17D yellow fever vaccine backbone	Age > 9 yrs.; increased risk of severe dengue in seronegative subjects; safe in seropositive people	Capeding, 2014 (29), Sabchareon, 2012 (28) Villar, 2015 (30) Flasche, 2019 (41) Halstead, 2021(16) Hadinegoro, 2015 (42) Sridhar, 2018 (43) Tully, 2021(25) Arredondo, 2018 (35)
	Tetravax; TV003/TV005	NIAID/NIH; Butantan; Merck (V181)	Phase 3	Attenuated DENV-1, -3, -4 with DENV-2/4 chimera backbone	Well-tolerated. Balanced immune responses, no ADE; single dosing. AEs: mild rash	Whitehead, 2017 (44) Kirkpatrick, 2015 (45)
	TAK-003; DENVax	Takeda; Inviragen	Phase 3	DENV-2 backbone with DENV-1, -3 & -4 substitutions	Immunogenic and well-tolerated in clinical studies, regardless of age or serostatus, safety profile analysis pending	Sirivichayakul, 2016 (46)
	TDEN F17/F19 (TDEN-LAV)	Walter Reed Army Institute of Research (WRAIR) and GSK	Phase 2 (stopped)	Tetravalent attenuated DENV-1-4	Safe, well-tolerated, immunogenic but more reactogenicity and unequal immune responses	Thomas, 2013 (47) Bauer, 2015 (48)

Vaccine Type	Vaccine Name	Developer	Current Stage	Strategy	Key Clinical Outcome	Ref
Inactivated	TDEN-PIV Tetravalent Dengue Purified Inactivated vaccine	GSK, WRAIR, and Oswaldo Cruz Foundation (Fiocruz)	Phase 1 (Stopped at Phase 1)	formalin-inactivated tetravalent with AS03 adjuvant	Good safety and immunogenic in naive and seropositive individuals. No risk of secondary dengue (not live vaccine), balanced immunological response	Schmidt, 2017 (49) Diaz, 2020 (50)
Recombinant Subunit portion of E protein	DEN-80E (V180)	GSK, Fiocruz, WRAIR. Merck	Phase 1 (Stopped at Phase 1)	recombinant portion of envelop protein	Induced immune responses against all DENV serotypes, decreasing likelihood of ADE effect.	Coller,2011 (51) Manoff,2015 (52) Precioso,2015 (53)
Nucleic acid (DNA) prM and E proteins	TVDV (Tetravalent dengue vaccine)	U.S. Naval Medical Research Center	Phase 1	Recombinant plasmid vector encoding prM/E proteins	Lack of immunogenicity. May need to test with adjuvant.	Beckett, 2010 (54) Danko, 2018 (55)
	D1ME100	US Naval Medical Research Center	Phase 1	recombinant plasmid vector encoding prM/E	No neutralizing antibody response detected. Need dose-escalation trial or add adjuvant.	Kochel, 2000 (56)

During the clinical trials, the tetravalent vaccine was found to have a vaccine efficacy of about 60% against developing dengue, and 67-80% efficacy in preventing hospitalization due to severe Dengue (61) which varied with the age of the recipient (63). In 2015, the WHO Strategic Advisory Group of Experts on Immunization (SAGE) Working group approved the use of Dengvaxia in dengue endemic areas, defined as regions with a seroprevalence of >70% in children. The vaccine was licensed initially in the Philippines, Mexico, and Brazil, and later licensed in a total of 20 countries (7, 64).

In 2017, the manufacturer reported that there were increased hospitalizations noted among children less than age nine years, two years after the first of the three-dose Dengvaxia vaccinations during the follow-up to the Phase 3 clinical trials. By the time that the increased hospitalizations had been reported, the Philippines government had vaccinated approximately 880,000 school children as part of a public health immunization initiative (64), the National Dengue Prevention and Control Program (7).

The increased number of hospitalizations were thought to be attributable to breakthrough dengue infections (due to the low vaccine efficacy of 30.2% reported in the Phase 2b trials, and ~60% in the Phase 3 trials), and not due to antibody-dependent enhancement (41). During the clinical trials, Sanofi used IgG/IgM ELISA testing on a small subset — less than 12% (64)— of subjects immunized to estimate the incidence of seronegative individuals prior to vaccination. They also relied on the population seroprevalence estimates being greater than 70% in the trial areas, as recommended by the WHO, rather than individually testing subjects. In 2018, Sanofi developed a new immunologic test, which measured dengue specific, anti-NS1 antibodies (43) which only could come from a prior dengue exposure since the NS1 proteins in the vaccine came from the 17D yellow fever backbone containing the non-structural coding regions. In addition, although dengue was reported to be the leading cause of hospitalization among children in the Philippines (65), and the dengue seropositivity of people aged 9-45 years old in Thailand was 86.5% (66), the estimated seropositivity among Filipino children was ~90% (59), the actual dengue seropositivity among Filipino children may have been less than the SAGE recommended threshold of greater than 70% (Eileen P Kelly, PhD, WRAIR, 13 November 2021, personal communications), and at least 10% of the 900,000 children vaccinated, or at least 90,00 children, who received Dengvaxia as part of the Philippine vaccination program would be seronegative without pre-testing for confirmation of prior dengue exposure (67).

There were 14 fatalities initially reported among those who had received at least one of the three-dose regimen of Dengvaxia, which were subsequently reviewed by the Dengue Investigative Task Force in the Philippines, and subsequently reviewed by the WHO Global Advisory Committee on Vaccine Safety (7), who found three confirmed cases of dengue shock syndrome following Dengvaxia immunization but indeterminant causality of the other cases regarding cause of death other than a temporal association (i.e., within eight days of vaccination) with the dengue vaccine. The Philippines Food and Drug Administration permanently suspended the vaccination program and withdrew its market licensure (68, 69). The WHO SAGE group revised its guidelines and recommended that the Dengvaxia vaccine only be given to children over the age of nine who lived in endemic areas with a seroprevalence of over 70%, or who were seropositive for a previous wildtype dengue infection (61, 70). These caveats were also imposed by the FDA in the United States who conditionally approved Dengvaxia on May 1, 2019, for use in endemic areas in people aged nine to 16 who were seropositive by laboratory testing for prior dengue infection (60, 69).

The Philippines Department of Justice indicted 14 government officials in February 2020 (71, 72), including the Health Secretary, the Principal Investigator, and six Sanofi executives for the deaths of children who died after receiving the Dengvaxia vaccine (73).

Reticence of parents to vaccinate their children because of the Dengvaxia safety concerns resulted in a marked decrease in measles and oral polio vaccinations in the Philippines (68) where childhood vaccination rates fell from 88% in 2014 to 55% in 2018 (74), with an attendant spike in measles cases (73, 75), and hesitancy to subsequently receive the COVID-19 vaccine (76). In 2019, the Philippines experienced a marked 97% increase in the number of cases of dengue. As environmental mosquito control measures have proven ineffective in controlling the prevalence of dengue, the Philippines Department of Health (DOH) have suggested that the ban on Dengvaxia be lifted to mitigate the incidence of dengue related hospitalizations and severe dengue (68). Dengvaxia remained approved for restricted use in people with prior seropositivity in an endemic area in 18 countries, including the US (59). Beginning in 1993, Sanofi spent an estimated US$1.5 billion developing a dengue vaccine. At the time of market approval in 2015, Dengvaxia was forecasted to bring in US$330 million by 2022, however 2016 sales were only €55 million in 2016, and only $4 million in 2017 (57, 77).

Cause of Dengvaxia related morbidity and mortality

If Dengvaxia contained antigens for the prM and E proteins of all four dengue serotypes, why would people who were immunized with the tetravalent dengue vaccine develop serious DHF or DSS with second infections? Wouldn't the tetravalent vaccine stimulate production of antibodies against all four serotypes contained in the vaccine? Although the Dengvaxia tetravalent vaccine contains prM and E codon regions from DENV-1, -2, -3 and -4 serotypes, it has been found that antibodies to the DENV-4 prM and E proteins predominate (3). These antibodies effectively neutralize DENV-4 viruses but are non-neutralizing for other serotypes. These non-neutralizing antibodies are thought to cause antibody-dependent enhancement (ADE), when the partial cross-reactivity wanes after two to three years. The preferential titers of DENV-4 despite the exposure to all four serotypes is due to the phenomenon of *viral interference* (3), seen when multiple strains were present in the same vaccine, resulting in non-neutralizing Abs against DENV-1, -2 and -3 reinfections. These non-neutralizing antibodies enhanced viral entry into the host cells and increased viral replication leading to higher viremia and severe dengue symptoms. This was seen during the clinical program in the Philippines where cases of severe dengue and hospitalizations increased two years after first vaccination with Dengvaxia. This was the likely cause of the increased numbers of hospitalizations and deaths two years after initial vaccination with Dengvaxia in the Philippines vaccination program (3), and the preferential production of anti-DENV-4 antibodies with non-neutralizing antibodies to the other three serotypes would account for the higher risk of dengue related hospitalizations in seronegative people immunized with Dengvaxia, 1.87% hospitalization for the placebo group versus 3.06% for the Dengvaxia group (43, 77).

Limitations

Limitation of the systematic literature review included the unavailability to access 36 of the articles via the University Library (see Figure 4 PRIMSA flow chart). Limitations of the studies reviewed:

1. Actual seroprevalence rates in endemic areas varied by geographic regions, differences between urban and rural incidence, age of the

population, and vary by year. There were few controlled studies of seroprevalence despite the WHO recommendations that Dengvaxia only be used in areas where the seroprevalence rate was above 70%.

2. Sanofi extrapolated the seropositive rate in the early Phase 3 trials by measuring anti-DENV IgG levels by ELISA on a small subset of subjects, however this test did not discriminate between prior dengue exposure or vaccination, and this test could produce false positives due to cross-reactivity with other flavivirus antibodies e.g., Zika, West Nile, or yellow fever, which often were endemic in the same areas. Sanofi later developed a more specific anti-DENV-NS1 test which would only be positive with prior dengue exposure.
3. Variations in the case definition of confirmed cases of dengue between the WHO and the CDC definitions, and the requirement to confirm cases with either the less specific ELISA IgG/IgM test or the more specific Plaque Reduction Neutralization Test (PRNT) was added by the WHO two years after the initial approval in 2015. The US FDA made laboratory confirmation a condition of approval of the Biologic License Application. Some of the severe cases were not considered to be vaccine related because of missing lab confirmation.
4. Potential under-reporting of cases of dengue infection or severe dengue due to the requirement to use either RT-PCR to detect dengue viral antigens in acute cases, or PRNT to detect anti-DENV neutralizing antibodies which are more difficult than the less sensitive rapid antigen test or ELISA for IgM/IgG (77). Reporting of adverse events during clinical trials is required by US Federal law at 21CFR312.25 (78), the International Committee on Harmonisation guidance ICH E2A (78) and by the European Medicines Agency (EMA) (79). Although Sanofi conducted both active and sentinel surveillance during post-marketing vaccination programs, the actual number of cases of confirmed severe dengue and deaths causally related to vaccination is likely to have been under-reported. Undurraga et al. (80) compared passive surveillance reporting of symptomatic dengue cases to active surveillance in a prospective cohort study with laboratory testing diagnostic confirmation and found underreporting of symptomatic cases by 4.7-fold and estimated that dengue cases in the Philippines were nearly 800,000 cases annually, rather than the 170,000 cases officially reported by the Philippines Department of Health (80).

5. There was no documentation of a correlation between Nab titers determined by PRNT and protection against dengue in the efficacy studies. Sanofi used antibody titers as a surrogate endpoint in lieu of tracking dengue breakthrough infections. Long-term (> 5 year) follow-up of the clinical trials is being done to track the real-world effectiveness of the dengue vaccine.
6. A complete pharmacovigilance (PV) safety analysis could not be conducted to determine the actual number of vaccine-related adverse and serious adverse events, therefore the documents submitted by Sanofi to the US FDA and the EMA for market approval, along with the package insert, company core data sheet in the public domain and the PV Assessment summary conducted by the FDA were used. Based on the data reviewed by the regulatory agencies that approved Dengvaxia, there did not appear to be a safety signal which would preclude approval. The FDA reported that there were 51 deaths reported worldwide during the post-marketing period from December 2015 through the date of the FDA BLA submission, of which 46 occurred in the Philippines. Of that number, only 10 met the criteria for laboratory confirmed severe dengue, and only 3 of those were confirmed by the FDA. It cannot be determined if the clinical and laboratory records were more complete if there would have been more confirmed cases. Nonetheless, Dengvaxia was conditionally approved by the FDA in 2019 only for ages 9-16 years old, living in endemic areas and with laboratory confirmed seropositive tests.

Recommendations

It is known that severe dengue occurs after a second infection with a different serotype from the first dengue exposure, at least 2-3 years after the first infection. The cases of severe dengue requiring hospitalization or death following Dengvaxia were thought to be due to antibody-dependent enhancement, not due to breakthrough secondary dengue due to ineffective vaccine efficacy from Dengvaxia (16, 17). Prior dengue infection is required by both the FDA and EMA for use of Dengvaxia with lab confirmation of prior dengue exposure before vaccination to prevent development of non-neutralizing antibodies which would cause ADE. The FDA and EMA now recommend individual testing for dengue antibodies before vaccination with

Dengvaxia, rather than relying on population seroprevalence rates and patient memory.

The ADE phenomenon more likely occurs with live attenuated virus vaccines, such as Dengvaxia and the 17D strain yellow fever vaccine (81). The prM and E proteins also are known to cause more non-neutralizing antibodies and higher rates of ADE than other regions of the dengue genome (3). There are eight other dengue vaccine candidates in various stages of clinical development, and the two that are in late Phase 3 do not have ADE phenomenon during clinical trials, and do not target the PrM or E proteins.

Conclusion

The only currently approved dengue vaccine, Dengvaxia is indicated for people aged 9 to 16 with documented prior exposure to dengue infection who are in an endemic area, per the U.S. CDC (8), or aged 9 to 45 years with a prior exposure to dengue living in an endemic area with a seroprevalence of greater than 70%, according to the WHO guidelines (82). There is difficulty in accurately assessing the seroprevalence rates in endemic areas, and the U.S. CDC (8) recommends that laboratory testing be done to confirm seropositive status prior to vaccination, rather than reliance on patients' memory of prior exposure (66). Dengvaxia should only be used in seropositive individuals and produces higher DENV-4 Abs than the other three serotypes. The WHO (83) recommended developing a vaccine that produced long-lasting immunity to all four serotypes without viral interference to balance the immune response and low reactogenicity in subjects with and without prior dengue exposure. Clinical safety and efficacy results for the two live, attenuated vaccine candidates currently in Phase 3 trials, as well as the four other dengue vaccine candidates is needed to assure that a safe and effective vaccine is available irrespective of prior dengue exposure, particularly since prior laboratory testing for dengue seropositivity is impractical and costly in most of the countries where dengue is hyperendemic.

Acknowledgments

The senior author sadly passed away on January 9th, 2023, he has served as the senior Medical Monitor on the Phase 1 and 2 trials of TV-003/005 conducted by the Johns Hopkins Bloomberg School of Public Health in his position as Director of the Clinical Safety Office for the vaccine sponsor, National Institute for Allergy and Infectious Diseases, NIH. The Author has also served as the Executive Director of Vaccine Clinical Safety and Risk Management for Merck, Sharpe and Dohme, although he was not involved with the development or review of V-180 or V-181(TetraVax).

References

[1] Gubler DJ, Ooi EE, Vasudevan S, Farrar J. Dengue and dengue hemorrhagic fever (2nd edition). Wallingford: CABI 2014. URL: https://www.cabdirect.org/globalhealth/abstract/20143309279.

[2] Gwee XWS, Chua PEY, Pang J. Global dengue importation: A systematic review. BMC Infect Dis 2021;21(1):1078.

[3] Shuklan R, Ramasamy V, Shanmugam RK, Ahuja R, Khanna N. Antibody-dependent enhancement: A challenge for developing a safe Dengue vaccine. Front Cell Infect Microbiol 2020;10:572681.

[4] Harapan H, Michie A, Sasmono RT, Imrie A. Dengue: A minireview. Viruses 2020;12(8):829.

[5] World Health Organization, UNICEF, UNDP, World Bank. Global vector control response 2017-2030. Geneva: World Health Organization, 2017.

[6] World Health Organization. Guidelines for the production and quality control of candidate tetravalent dengue virus vaccines (live). Geneva: World Health Organization, 2006.

[7] World Health Organization. Safety of dengue vaccine in the Philippines. Geneva: World Health Organization, 2018.

[8] Centers for Disease Control and Prevention. Dengue. Atlanta, GA: CDC; 2021 URL: https://www.cdc.gov/dengue/index.html.

[9] Fact sheet: Vector-borne diseases. World Health Organization; 2020 Mar 2. URL: https://www.who.int/news-room/fact-sheets/detail/vector-borne-diseases.

[10] Bowman LR, Donegan S, McCall PJ. Is Dengue Vector Control Deficient in Effectiveness or Evidence?: Systematic Review and Meta-analysis. PLoS Negl Trop Dis 2016;10(3): e0004551.

[11] World Health Organization. Dengue increase likely during rainy season: WHO warns. Geneva: World Health Organization, 2019.

[12] Messina JP, Brady OJ, Golding N, Kraemer MUG, Wint GRW, Ray SE, et al. The current and future global distribution and population at risk of dengue. Nat Microbiol 2019;4(9): 9. URL: https://geneticliteracyproject.org/2022/03/11/2-5-billion-gene-altered-mosquitoes-designed-to-end-spread-of-zika-dengue-and-malaria-to-be-released-in-two-year-experiment-in-california-and-florida-fda-decides/.

[13] Mustafa MS, Rasotgi V, Jain S, Gupta V. Discovery of fifth serotype of dengue virus (DENV-5): A new public health dilemma in dengue control. Med J Armed Forces India 2015;71(1):67–70.

[14] Taylor-Robinson AW. A putative fifth serotype of Dengue—Potential implications for diagnosis, therapy and vaccine design. Int J Clin Med Microbiol 2016;1(101): IJCMM.

[15] Sabin AB. Research on Dengue during World War II. Am J Trop Med 1952;1(1):30–50.

[16] Halstead SB. Vaccine-associated enhanced viral disease: Implications for viral vaccine development. BioDrugs 2021;35(5):505–15.

[17] Guzman MG, Alvarez M, Halstead SB. Secondary infection as a risk factor for dengue hemorrhagic fever/dengue shock syndrome: An historical perspective and role of antibody-dependent enhancement of infection. Arch Virol 2013;158(7): 1445-59.

[18] Ulrich H, Pillat MM, Tárnok A. Dengue Fever, COVID-19 (SARS-CoV-2), and antibody-dependent enhancement (ADE): A perspective. Cytometry A 2020;97(7): 662–7.

[19] Halstead SB, O'Rourke EJ. Editorial response: Resuscitation of patients with Dengue hemorrhagic fever/Dengue shock syndrome. Clin Infect Dis 1999;29(4): 795-6.

[20] Lacy ER. Dengue in Grenada: Disease surveillance and vector assessment. Master's thesis. Grenada: St George's University, 1998.

[21] Page MJ, McKenzie JE, Bossuyt PM, Boutron I, Hoffmann TC, Mulrow CD, et al. The PRISMA 2020 statement: An updated guideline for reporting systematic reviews. BMJ 2021;372:n71.

[22] Lang J. Recent progress on Sanofi Pasteur's dengue vaccine candidate. J Clin Virol 2009;46:S20–4.

[23] Thomas SJ, Yoon IK. A review of Dengvaxia®: development to deployment. Hum Vaccin Immunother 2019;15(10):2295-314. DOI: 10.1080/21645515.2019.1658503.

[24] Guy B, Briand O, Lang J, Saville M, Jackson N. Development of the Sanofi Pasteur tetravalent Dengue vaccine: One more step forward. Vaccine 2015;33(50):7100-11.

[25] Tully D, Griffiths CL. Dengvaxia: The world's first vaccine for prevention of secondary dengue. Ther Adv Vaccines Immunother 2021;9:25151355211015839.

[26] Guy B. Immunogenicity of Sanofi Pasteur tetravalent dengue vaccine. J Clin Virol 2009;46:S16-9.

[27] Tricou V, Sáez-Llorens X, Yu D, Rivera L, Jimeno J, Villarreal AC, et al. Safety and immunogenicity of a tetravalent dengue vaccine in children aged 2-17 years: A randomised, placebo-controlled, phase 2 trial. Lancet 2020;395(10234):1434-43.

[28] Sabchareon A, Wallace D, Sirivichayakul C, Limkittikul K, Chanthavanich P, Suvannadabba S, et al. Protective efficacy of the recombinant, live-attenuated, CYD tetravalent dengue vaccine in Thai schoolchildren: A randomised, controlled phase 2b trial. Lancet 2012;380(9853):1559-67.

[29] Capeding MR, Tran NH, Hadinegoro SRS, Ismail HIHJM, Chotpitayasunondh T, Chua MN, et al. Clinical efficacy and safety of a novel tetravalent dengue vaccine

in healthy children in Asia: A phase 3, randomised, observer-masked, placebo-controlled trial. Lancet 2014;384(9951):1358-65.

[30] Villar L, Dayan GH, Arredondo-García JL, Rivera DM, Cunha R, Deseda C, et al. Efficacy of a tetravalent dengue vaccine in children in Latin America. N Engl J Med 2015;372(2):113-23.

[31] Hombach J. Guidelines for clinical trials of dengue vaccine in endemic areas. J Clin Virol 2009;46:S7-9.

[32] Letson GW. Dengue surveillance in preparation for field vaccine trials. J Clin Virol 2009;46:S10-2.

[33] Rodriguez-Barraquer I, Mier-y-Teran-Romero L, Burke DS, Cummings DAT. Challenges in the interpretation of dengue vaccine trial results. PLoS Negl Trop Dis 2013;7(8):e2126.

[34] Wilder-Smith A. Dengue vaccine development: Status and future. Bundesgesundheitsblatt Gesundheitsforschung Gesundheitsschutz 2019;63(1):40–4.

[35] Zambrano B, Noriega F, Dayan GH, Rivera DM, Arredondo JL, Reynales H, et al. Zika and Dengue interactions in the context of a large Dengue vaccine clinical trial in Latin America. Am J Trop Med 2021;104(1):136-44.

[36] Ponndorf D, Meshcheriakova Y, Thuenemann EC, Dobon Alonso A, Overman R, et al. Plant-made dengue virus-like particles produced by co-expression of structural and non-structural proteins induce a humoral immune response in mice. Plant Biotechnol J 2021;19(4):745-56.

[37] McKain S. The prevalence of Dengue and its serotypes in Grenada: A five-year retrospective study. Master's thesis. Grenada: St George's University, 2015.

[38] Panagos A. A Seroprevalence and K.A.P survey of Dengue fever in Grenada. Master's thesis. Grenada: St George's University, 1996.

[39] Pulim S. Dengue in St George's University 1997-1998. Master's thesis. Grenada: St George's University, 2003.

[40] Schiøler KL. Dengue transmission and surveillance in a small-island setting: A case study from Grenada. Dissertation. Grenada: St George's University, 2006.

[41] Flasche S, Wilder-Smith A, Hombach J, Smith PG. Estimating the proportion of vaccine-induced hospitalized dengue cases among Dengvaxia vaccinees in the Philippines. Wellcome Open Res 2019;4:165.

[42] Hadinegoro SR, Arredondo-García JL, Capeding MR, Deseda C, Chotpitayasunondh T, Dietze R, et al. Efficacy and long-term safety of a Dengue vaccine in regions of endemic disease. N Engl J Med 2015;373(13):1195-206.

[43] Sridhar S, Luedtke A, Langevin E, Zhu M, Bonaparte M, Machabert T, et al. Effect of Dengue Serostatus on Dengue Vaccine Safety and Efficacy. N Engl J Med 2018;379(4):327-40.

[44] Whitehead SS, Durbin AP, Pierce KK, Elwood D, McElvany BD, Fraser EA, et al. In a randomized trial, the live attenuated tetravalent dengue vaccine TV003 is well-tolerated and highly immunogenic in subjects with flavivirus exposure prior to vaccination. PLoS Negl Trop Dis 2017;11(5):0005584.

[45] Kirkpatrick BD, Durbin AP, Pierce KK, Carmolli MP, Tibery CM, Grier PL, et al. Robust and balanced immune responses to all 4 Dengue virus serotypes following

administration of a single dose of a live aqttenuated tetravalent Dengue vaccine to healthy, Flavivirus-Naive adults. J Infect Dis 2015;212(5):702-10.

[46] Sirivichayakul C, Barranco-Santana EA, Esquilin-Rivera I, Oh HML, Raanan M, Sariol CA, et al. Safety and immunogenicity of a tetravalent Dengue vaccine candidate in healthy children and adults in Dengue-endemic regions: A randomized, placebo-controlled Phase 2 Study. J Infect Dis 2016;213(10):1562-72.

[47] Thomas SJ, Eckels KH, Carletti I, De La Barrera R, Dessy F, Fernandez S, et al. A phase II, randomized, safety and immunogenicity study of a re-derived, live-attenuated Dengue virus vaccine in healthy adults. Am J Trop Med 2013;88(1):73–88.

[48] Bauer K, Esquilin IO, Cornier AS, Thomas SJ, Quintero Del Rio AI, Bertran-Pasarell J, et al. A phase II, randomized, safety and immunogenicity trial of a re-derived, live-attenuated Dengue virus vaccine in healthy children and adults living in Puerto Rico. Am J Trop Med Hyg 2015;93(3):441-53.

[49] Schmidt AC, Lin L, Martinez LJ, Ruck RC, Eckels KH, Collard A, et al. Phase 1 randomized study of a tetravalent Dengue purified inactivated vaccine in healthy adults in the United States. Am J Trop Med Hyg 2017;96(6):1325-37.

[50] Diaz C, Lin L, Martinez LJ, Eckels KH, Campos M, Jarman RG, et al. Phase I randomized study of a tetravalent Dengue purified inactivated vaccine in healthy adults from Puerto Rico. Am J Trop Med Hyg 2018;98(5):1435-43.

[51] Coller BA. G Clements, DE, Bett AJ, Sagar SL, Ter Meulen JH. The development of recombinant subunit envelope-based vaccines to protect against dengue virus induced disease. Vaccine 2011;29(42):7267-75.

[52] Manoff SB, George SL, Bett AJ, Yelmene ML, Dhanasekaran G, Eggemeyer L, et al. Preclinical and clinical development of a dengue recombinant subunit vaccine. Vaccine 2015;33(50):7126-34.

[53] Precioso AR, Palacios R, Thomé B, Mondini G, Braga P, Kalil J. Clinical evaluation strategies for a live attenuated tetravalent dengue vaccine. Vaccine 2015;33(50):7121-5.

[54] Beckett CG, Tjaden J, Burgess T, Danko JR, Tamminga C, Simmons M, et al. Evaluation of a prototype dengue-1 DNA vaccine in a Phase 1 clinical trial. Vaccine 2010;29(5):960-8.

[55] Danko JR, Kochel T, Teneza-Mora N, Luke TC, Raviprakash K, Sun P, et al. Safety and immunogenicity of a tetravalent Dengue DNA vaccine administered with a cationic lipid-based adjuvant in a phase 1 clinical trial. Am J Trop Med Hyg 2018;98(3):849-56.

[56] Kochel TJ, Raviprakash K, Hayes CG, Watts DM, Russell KL, Gozalo AS, et al. A Dengue virus serotype-1 DNA vaccine induces virus neutralizing antibodies and provides protection from viral challenge in Aotus monkeys. Vaccine 2000;18(27): 3166-73.

[57] Drugood. Observing the difficult development course of Dengue fever vaccine from the rise and fall of Dengvaxia. Drugood 2018 May 05. URL: https://web.archive.org/web/20200929205944/http://www.drugood.com/2018/05/05/observing-the-difficult-development-course-of-dengue-fever-vaccine-from-the-rise-and-fall-of-dengvaxia/.

[58] Halstead SB. Safety issues from a phase 3 clinical trial of a live-attenuated chimeric yellow fever tetravalent dengue vaccine. Hum Vaccin Immunother 2018;14(9): 2158-62.

[59] Eng KF. What went wrong with the breakthrough dengue vaccine? New York: TED Fellows; 2018. https://fellowsblog.ted.com/what-went-wrong-with-the-break through-dengue-vaccine-cf8519cb90c8.

[60] LeBlanc R. Clinical review memo—DENGVAXIA biological license application. Washington, DC: Division of Vaccines and Related Product Applications (CBER/FDA); 2018. URL: https://www.fda.gov/media/125480/download.

[61] Durbin AP. A Dengue vaccine. Cell 2016;166(1):1.

[62] Hajj Hussein I, Chams N, Chams S, El Sayegh S, Badran R, Raad M, et al. Vaccines through centuries: Major cornerstones of global health. Front Public Health 2015;3:269.

[63] World Health Organization. Dengue Bulletin, Volume 41. Geneva: World Health Organization, 2020.

[64] Halstead SB, Katzelnick LC, Russell PK, Markoff L, Aguiar M, Dans LR, et al. Ethics of a partially effective dengue vaccine: Lessons from the Philippines. Vaccine 2022;38(35):5572-6.

[65] Oishi K, Mapua CA, Carlos CC, Cinco-Abanes MTDD, Saito M, Inoue S, et al. Dengue and other febrile illnesses among children in the Philippines. Dengue Bull 2006;30:9.

[66] Buddhari D, Anderson KB, Gromowski GD, Jarman RG, Iamsirithaworn S, Thaisomboonsuk B, et al. Correlation between reported dengue illness history and seropositivity in rural Thailand. PLoS Negl Trop Dis 2021;15(6):0009459.

[67] Fatima K, Syed NI. Dengvaxia controversy: Impact on vaccine hesitancy. J Glob Health 2018;8(2):020312.

[68] Fonbuena C. Hundreds of children die in Philippine Dengue epidemic as local action urged. Guardian 2019 Sep 12. URL: https://www.theguardian.com/global-development/2019/sep/12/hundreds-of-children-die-in-philippine-dengue-epidemic-as-local-action-urged.

[69] TrialSite Staff. The lasting impact of the Dengue vaccine controversy in the Philippines. Trial Site News 2021 Sep 27. URL: https://www.trialsitenews.com/a/the-lasting-impact-of-the-dengue-vaccine-controversy-in-the-philippines.

[70] Nelson C. CYD-TDV – Dengvaxia® – Sanofi Pasteur clinical update. Arboviruses: A global public health threat, Les Pensières Center for Global Health, Veyrier-du-Lac (France). Sanofi Pasteur, 2018. URL: https://www.fondation-merieux.org/wp-content/uploads/2018/01/arboviruses-2018-christopher-nelson.pdf.

[71] Macairan E. DOJ indicts Garin, 9 others for Dengvaxia deaths. Manila (Philippines). Philippine Star 2019 Mar 02. URL: https://www.philstar.com/headlines/2019/03/02/1898019/doj-indicts-garin-9-others-dengvaxia-deaths.

[72] Ramirez R. DOJ indicts Garin, others over Dengvaxia. Philstar Global 2020 Feb 22. URL: https://www.philstar.com/headlines/2020/02/22/1995119/doj-indicts-garin-others-over-dengvaxia.

[73] Doucleff M. Dengue vaccine controversy in the Philippines. Washington, DC: NPR 2019 May 02. URL: https://www.npr.org/2019/05/02/719366831/dengue-vaccine-controversy-in-the-philippines.
[74] Alfonso C, Dayrit M, Mendoza R, Ong M. From Dengvaxia to Sinovac: Vaccine hesitancy in the Philippines. Diplomat 2021 Mar 08. URL: https://thediplomat.com/2021/03/from-dengvaxia-to-sinovac-vaccine-hesitancy-in-the-philippines/.
[75] International Federation of the Red Cross and Red Crescent Societies. Operations update Philippines: Re-emergence of vaccine preventable diseases – Measles outbreak. Geneva: IFRC, 2020. URL: https://reliefweb.int/sites/reliefweb.int/files/resources/MDRPH03212m_measles.pdf.
[76] Lasco G, Yu VG. Communicating COVID-19 vaccines: Lessons from the dengue vaccine controversy in the Philippines. BMJ Glob Health 2021;6(3):005422.
[77] Wood L. Global Dengue vaccines disease market analysis report 2021-2022: Dengvaxia's uptake will remain minimal before pipeline rivals launch. Dublin: Research and Markets, 2021. URL: https://finance.yahoo.com/news/global-dengue-vaccines-disease-market-084800202.html.
[78] US Food and Drug Administration. Silver Spring, MD: Department of Health and Human Services, 2022. Code of Federal Regulations Title 21 Sect. 312.25, Investigational new drug safety reporting. URL: https://www.accessdata.fda.gov/scripts/cdrh/cfdocs/cfCFR/CFRSearch.cfm?fr=312.32.
[79] EMA. ICH E 2 A clinical safety data management: Definitions and standards for expedited reporting. Amsterdam: EMA, 1995. URL: https://www.ema.europa.eu/en/ich-e2a-clinical-safety-data-management-definitions-standards-expedited-reporting.
[80] Undurraga EA, Edillo FE, Erasmo JNV, Alera MTP, Yoon I-K, Largo FM, et al. Disease burden of Dengue in the Philippines: Adjusting for underreporting by comparing active and passive Dengue surveillance in Punta Princesa, Cebu City. Am J Trop Med 2017;96(4):887-98.
[81] Izmirly AM, Alturki SO, Alturki SO, Connors J, Haddad EK. Challenges in Dengue vaccines development: Pre-existing infections and cross-reactivity. Front Immunol 2020; 11:1055.
[82] World Health Organization. Vaccines and immunization: Dengue. Geneva: World Health Organization, 2018. URL: https://www.who.int/news-room/questions-and-answers/item/dengue-vaccines.
[83] World Health Organization. Dengue guidelines for diagnosis, treatment, prevention and control: new edition. Geneva: World Health Organization, 2009.

Chapter 13

Workplace safety and occupational health hazards at the General Hospital in Grenada, West Indies

Nesta Edwards, MPH
Anthony La, BA
Emmanuel O Keku, MD, MA, MSPH
and Lindonne Telesford*, MSPH, DrPH
School of Medicine, Department of Public Health and Preventive Medicine,
St George's University, St George, Grenada, West Indies

Abstract

Healthcare workers often function in unsafe conditions, exposed to chemical, physical, biological, ergonomic, and psychosocial hazards. The study identifies workers' perceptions of occupational hazards at a hospital in Grenada prior to and during the COVID-19 pandemic. A retrospective mixed-method pilot study was administered to ten workers at the General Hospital in 2022. The study included a survey followed by face-to-face interviews. Convenience sampling was used to recruit nurses, orderlies, medical waste handlers, and laboratory technicians. The themes derived from responses were poor work culture, poor workplace design, staff shortage, low level of motivation, lack of ergonomically designed spaces, inadequate personal protective equipment, and insufficient planning for risk remediation. Psychological,

* Corresponding Author's Email: ltelesfor@sgu.edu; Dr. Lindonne Telesford, MSPH, DrPH, Associate Professor, School of Medicine, St George's University, Department of Public Health, and Preventive Medicine, PO Box 7, St George, Grenada, West Indies.

In: Public Health
Editors: Emmanuel O Keku and Joav Merrick
ISBN: 979-8-89113-083-8

biological, and physical hazards were found to increase during the COVID-19 pandemic period. The result of the study is indicative of occupational health risk and impacts on workers at the hospital. This information is useful to guide policy to improve safety, minimize hazards, and improve the delivery of healthcare services in Grenada.

Keywords: COVID-19, Grenada, occupational safety, physical hazards, biological hazards, psychosocial hazards, personal protective equipment, hospital environment, ergonomic

Introduction

Hospitals are comparably one of the most high-risk working environments. People who work in hospitals often experience unsafe working conditions, work-generated injuries, and the exponential risk of exposure to life-threatening diseases. In 2019, hospitals in the United States received reports of 221,400 workplace injuries and illnesses (1).

Occupational diseases can have significant impacts not only on workers' health and well-being but also productivity. Studies from high-and low-income countries found that healthcare workers were often exposed to biological, chemical, physical, ergonomic, and psychosocial hazards in the work environments (2-5). Latin American countries and the Caribbean region recorded one of the highest fatality rates due to hazardous work-related exposures (6, 7) which illustrates a gap in occupational safety and health (OSH) standards.

OSH are grossly ignored, largely, in poorer and developing countries. Studies revealed that the COVID-19 pandemic further resulted in decline in the application of OSH practices in healthcare settings (8, 9). Working conditions in the healthcare sector in both high- and low-income countries were affected and had adverse consequences for the quality of health care delivery, workers' productivity, and inherently, economics due to the COVID-19 pandemic. Several institutions have and continue to implement measures to eliminate or control occupational health risks in healthcare settings. Nonetheless, studies are needed to create a better understanding of the factors that implicate workers' health in respective settings and to improve the occupational environment.

The study was conducted to investigate workers' perceptions of occupational hazards at a hospital in Grenada prior to and during the COVID-

19 pandemic. Three questions were addressed relating to the General Hospital: (1) What types of hazards were employees exposed to in specific work activities? (2) What factors were contributing to occupational health hazards? (3) What occupational safety and health challenges were experienced prior to and during the COVID-19 pandemic?

The study provides critical insights on OSH needs to improve working conditions for employees in the health sector. The resilience of the health sector in epidemics and pandemics can be improved through strengthening occupational health systems that protect workers.

Methods

A retrospective qualitative mixed-methods study was conducted with information collected through a survey and face-to-face interviews with workers at the General Hospital in Grenada. Four groups of workers participated in the study in March to April 2022.

Participants were identified through convenience sampling and recruited based on the inclusion criteria. An invitation was extended to workers in the selected categories to participate. Twenty workers were available, of which ten gave written informed consent to participate. The inclusion criteria were male and female employees between 18 and 60 years working at the General Hospital for at least five years in the positions of either nurse, laboratory technician, medical waste handler, or orderly. Students, workers on leave, and workers not fluent in English were excluded from participating in the study.

The self-administered survey included ten close-ended questions on participants demographics, satisfaction with occupational safety measures, and experience with occupational accidents and injuries. Individual face-to-face interviews were conducted at the same location immediately after completing the survey, while ensuring adherence of COVID-19 protocols. Ten questions were asked with probing for approximately 40 minutes per participant. Each interview was recorded with permission from the participant. The recordings allowed for accurate transcription of the information. Handwritten notes were also taken by the interviewer. Codes were used to de-identify matching participants in the interviews. Participants shared their experiences relating to workplace safety and health hazards prior to and during the COVID-19 pandemic periods.

Data analysis

Data from completed surveys was recorded in a Microsoft Excel worksheet and imported into Epi Info version 7.2.4.0. to conduct descriptive analysis. Interview notes and recordings were transcribed by the investigator and common themes were identified. Transcriptions were carefully reviewed to extract significant statements that matched themes.

Ethical considerations

Ethical approval for the study was granted by the St George's University Institutional Review Board (IRB).

Results

The study participants included nurses, orderlies, medical waste handlers, and laboratory technicians employed at the General Hospital. Ten workers participated, inclusive of males and females, aged 26 to 50 years. Most of the participants were employed at the hospital for at least ten years. The participants completed education at university, secondary school, and primary school. Table 1 shows demographic information for the participants.

Table 1. Demographics of study participants

Characteristics	Study Group (N) = 10
Age Group (years)	
26-35	5
36-45	2
45-50	3
Gender	
Male	3
Female	7
Completion of Education	
University	3
Secondary School	3
Primary School	4
Work Tenure at the Hospital	
5–10 years	4
10 years +	6

Satisfaction with OHS measures at the General Hospital

Forty percent (40%) of the participants reported being satisfied with the current OSH measures at the General Hospital. Thirty percent (30%) stated that they were dissatisfied and 30% were neutral or unresponsive. Two of the participants who reported being satisfied with the current OSH measures had education lower than secondary level.

All participants reported that they were required to wear personal protective equipment (PPE) when carrying out work activities. Perceptions of safety were described as poor (30%) and moderate (50%). Twenty percent of the participants were neutral. Figure 1 shows participants' satisfaction with OSH measures at the General Hospital.

Half (50%) of the participants indicated they received an occupational injury before and/or during COVID-19 pandemic while working at the hospital. Limited knowledge on OSH (60%) and unavailable PPE (40%) were cited as the main causes of injuries and accidents. All participants indicated that they have been impacted by the COVID-19 pandemic at work. The mean rating for the extent to which participants were affected by COVID-19 was 7.9 on a scale of 1-10. The participants also stated that some OSH changes occurred during the COVID-19 pandemic, such as increase in PPE supplies and training in PPE use. Participants' responses to the hazards they experienced at the General Hospital were biological (100%), physical (80%), ergonomic (70%), and psychosocial (90%).

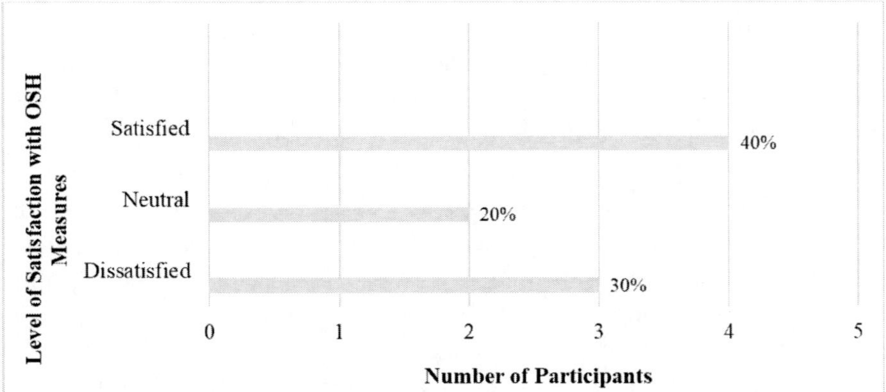

Figure 1. Level of satisfaction with OSH measures reported by workers at the General Hospital.

Qualitative analysis

Pre-COVID-19 period

Participants reported that several OSH challenges existed prior to the COVID-19 pandemic. Workers indicated that most of their health hazards were in relation to work design, safety practices, PPE availability, communication, and exposure to different hazards. The following themes and information were derived from the interviews:

Poor work culture

Despite training on safety practices, the participants reported several instances of near misses for needlestick injuries due to poor work practices, improper disposal, and negligence. None of the participants, however, reported receiving a needlestick injury.

Participant 4 stated, "There have been instances where doctors and even nurses struck needles into patients' mattresses or placed used needles on the lid of the sharp's containers." The participant further explained that the low nurse-patient ratio sometimes contributes to the occurrence of improper disposal of needles and that constantly having to worry about safety and health is mentally challenging and affects optimal job performance. Participant 4 also stated, "Although, these practices have gotten lesser over the past months, it's a matter of life and death."

Biological and physical hazards

Most of the participants reported being exposed to physical, biological, ergonomic, and psychological hazards while at work. Participants reported that they were at high risk of exposure to bloodborne pathogens from overflowing sharps container and needles found in patients' mattresses and bedsheets. Exposure to urine and blood was also reported as a hazard for health workers at the institution. Participants reported receiving cuts, bruises, and slips while assisting patients due to inadequate spacing or the type of equipment used. Storing, carrying, and removing hazardous materials like sharps, along with adjusting faulty patient beds have also been reported as hazardous for the workers at the hospital. Participant 1 stated, "The head nurses (sisters) have given gentle reminders to refrain from such unsafe practices, but it continues to happen." Participant 3 also stated, "I have never been spat on, but I saw it happen to my co-workers, I worry that a patient may attack me."

Psychosocial hazards

Long working hours, demanding work environment, burnout, fear of infection from bloodborne pathogens, verbal abuse from visitors, poor workplace design, non-compliance with health and safety protocols among colleagues, limited involvement of management, and inadequate spacing [to relax, eat, debrief] were the main psychosocial hazards reported by participants. Participate 6 explained, "Some visitors become verbally abusive when restricted to see their families or friends during the spike in COVID-19 patients at the General Hospital."

Inadequacy of personal protective equipment (PPE)

Most of the participants reported on PPE shortage which resulted in inadequate protection of workers on occasions. Participant 6 stated, "Sometimes we run out of gloves and work without because it may take weeks to get supplies. We also work with sub-standard quality gloves sometimes."

Lack of ergonomics designs

The participants reported that workers have an increased risk of injuries from lifting patients, moving, and handling equipment due to malfunctioning elevators, insufficient support staff, and differences in the level of knowledge on safe lifting among workers. Participant 4 stated, "We have not received any updated training in quite a while."

Poor workplace design

Participants reported on poorly ventilated rooms and not having sufficient shelves/stands to store items such as PPE, medical tools, and personal items. The lack of debriefing rooms, poorly designed fire emergency exits, and lack of changing rooms were also cited as workplace design issues. Participant 5 stated, "There were issues such as nonfunctional hand sanitizing dispensers and not having a handwashing sink in close proximity to disinfect their hands following their interaction with patients." Participant 2 stated, "We have leaking air conditioning unit, roofing issues, and where we take our lunch is very congested due to limited spacing." Participant 1 stated, "When roofing materials get wet, it soaks, fall to the floor and the leaking AC makes the floor wet and slippery from time to time and there is rarely any hazard sign to alert workers of a wet floor." The participant also stated, "There are no ramps/steps and exit doors in my department in case of a fire hazard." There were reports that the structure of certain wards can increase the possibility of spreading infectious diseases. Participant 6 stated, "It would be nice if separators are placed between the wards where highly sensitive cases are being treated."

COVID-19 pandemic challenges

Staffing shortage

Nurse-patient ratio was highlighted as a major contributor to psychological hazards at the hospital. Participants explained that the nurse-patient ratio is extremely unbalanced and exacerbated during the COVID-19 pandemic. The participants stated that the challenges of staff shortage at the hospital intensified when staff started contracting COVID-19, which resulted in a smaller workforce and added workload for workers on shift. Participant 1 explained that because some workers contracted COVID-19, other workers were challenged by longer working hours, low nurse-patient ratio, burnout and being fearful of losing coworkers to the disease. Participant 8 stated, "The nurse-patient ratio was very challenging and strenuous physically and psychologically during the major spike in COVID-19 cases because we must fill in the gaps for staff on sick-leave and multi-task for hours without short breaks. This, along with difficulty taking short breaks due to the patient's health conditions and demands, can be very stressful over prolonged periods."

Low levels of motivation

Workers' motivation was reported as higher before the COVID-19 pandemic. Participants stated their motivation fluctuated, especially during the initial phase of the pandemic. Participant 9 explained, "The conditions of the hospital have really motivated me to work harder and be more vigilant in order for me to feel safe but when COVID-19 came I had little motivation to work because I was afraid of getting infected and passing it to my family."

Insufficient planning, organizing and training

Some participants stated that weekly training increased due to the pandemic, especially on donning and doffing PPE and use of COVID-19 related diagnostic and treatment machinery. Participant 10 stated, "We have been asking for training, but none has been provided in the last two years."

Training was introduced during the COVID-19 pandemic to some participants on Mondays, Wednesdays, and Fridays; however, some staff members reported that it was extremely challenging to attend training sessions mostly for three reasons: 1) Staff shortage when other workers were on vacation and/or sick leave, 2) Training was sometimes held on leave days which disrupted rest and self-care routine for the workers and 3) Staff restricted to wards based on number of patients and needs. Participant 4 explained, "Despite all the training nurses have been receiving, unsafe needle disposal continues to exist which increases the risk of biological hazards." Participant 8 further stated, "My job is extremely sensitive; however, when I started, no formal training was given to me. I had to learn on my own or observe others. This can be bad if I am observing someone who is non-compliant to safety practices." Participant 10 also stated, "COVID- 19 has given me lots of training opportunities such as donning and doffing gloves and other PPE, importance of hygiene practices and consistency in adhering to workplace health protocols." Most of the participants expressed that training could be more effective if supervision improved, and penalties enforced for non-compliance. Many participants also stated that better communication between supervisors and subordinates can improve planning, organizing, and training at the General Hospital.

Suitability of PPE

All participants indicated that PPE was provided by the hospital. The workers reported that supplies of PPE increased during the COVID-19 pandemic. Apart from gloves, workers reported that aprons, face shield, goggles, and face masks were also available. However, most workers also stated that there were issues relating to PPE size, preference, comfort, effectiveness, and quality. Participant 7 stated, "I have always had issues getting gloves my size over the past 10 years."

Impact of COVID-19 pandemic

All participants reported that they were negatively impacted by COVID-19 pandemic at work. The main concerns reported were related to the level of preparedness of the General Hospital about spacing, resources, staffing, and security. Longer and unpredictable working hours, shorter breaks, and increased susceptibility to contracting and spreading COVID-19 to family were reported by most participants. In addition, participants expressed being psychologically affected because they were extremely fearful of losing their co-workers and infecting their families with COVID-19. Participants also reported feeling insecure due to insufficient security guards on the General Hospital compound. Participant 2 stated, "This resulted in COVID-19 patients violating hospital restrictions and mingling with patients from other wards." Participants stated that COVID-19 negatively influenced work procedures and practices, PPE supplies (gloves, face masks), and training in PPE use. Participant 3 stated that the General Hospital is more prepared should another wave of COVID-19 infections occur. All participants expressed that the General Hospital was unprepared for COVID-19, however, proactive measures were quickly adopted to effectively address the growing numbers of in-patients who were infected with the disease and other ailments. Participant 6 said, "This gave us a sense of hope!" Participant 9 also stated, "Although there is room for improvement, we feel more prepared to deal with health crises."

Discussion

This study revealed OSH hazards faced by nurses, lab technicians, medical waste handlers and orderlies at the General Hospital in Grenada. The study also provided insights on occupational health concerns experienced before and during the COVID-19 pandemic. The themes derived from responses were poor work culture, poor workplace design, staff shortage, low level of motivation, lack of ergonomically designed spaces, inadequate personal protective equipment, and insufficient planning for risk remediation. It is notable that some challenges existed in both periods, but with different frequency and intensity. For example, psychosocial hazards existed from pre-COVID-19 times, but were exacerbated during the COVID-19 pandemic.

Occupational safety and health standards challenges at the General Hospital were multifactorial and consistent with findings from across the globe. Studies from other countries show that knowledge, access to training, and enforcement of protocols, play an important role in ensuring safety in healthcare settings (10, 11) The working conditions of employees in hospital settings have an overall influence on their health and well-being (12), which in turn affects the quality of services provided by the workers (13). Ignoring the provision of OSH for healthcare workers can result in both short and long-term repercussions for national health care delivery and population health outcomes.

Our findings indicate that all study participants are potentially at risk of biological, physical, ergonomic, and psychosocial hazards due to poorly enforced OSH measures. The most frequently reported hazards were biological and psychosocial, attributed to lack of accountability for proper usage of sharps containers, staff shortage, and burnout from long working hours and a demanding work environment. The current study finding is consistent with a study conducted in North America which illustrated that needlestick injuries are mainly attributed to unsafe practices and negligence in healthcare professionals (14). This implies that following appropriate needlestick protocols in hospitals can aid in prevention and reduction of needlestick injuries. Increasing surveillance and having practical training sessions on handling and disposing needles should be prioritized. Some researchers have identified that in many cases needlestick injuries are underreported (15). Other studies also showed that nurses were at a higher risk of needlestick injuries compared to other workers (16). Job title, sex, lack of experience, workload, poor knowledge of bloodborne pathogens diseases and improper use of PPE were found to be some of the main reasons for needlestick injuries in hospital settings in high- and low-income countries (17, 18).

Attention should be given to addressing these factors to reduce occupational accidents and injuries in the hospital and other health care settings. Programs should be developed for regular re-training of health workers and monitoring the application of protocols. Several studies also highlighted the role of considering workers' PPE preferences in reducing and preventing unsafe practices and exposure to OSH hazards (19-22). Future studies should also examine whether there were associations between participants' work tenure and experiencing accidents and injuries in the hospital. These studies can provide critical evidence to support policies related to training, re-training, and other capacity development of workers. This study found elevated psychosocial hazards during the COVID-19 pandemic resulting from increased demands on health care with longer and unpredictable working hours. Staff shortage became a major issue as more healthcare workers were infected with COVID-19, increasing the workload of workers. Participants disclosed that they were extremely fearful of contracting the novel coronavirus and transmitting infection to their families. Psychosocial hazards can lead to serious mental health problems for healthcare workers (23). On the other hand, a safe work environment can contribute to improved quality of patient care, job satisfaction, performance, efficiency, and effectiveness (24). A supportive hospital administration may result in increased motivation, performance, and influence better communicative channels for reporting workplace issues. Support from health administrators and supervisors may also strengthen relationships and adherence to workplace policies which is one of the pillars for a healthy working environment. Lack of support from health administrators and excessive workload exacerbate mental health issues in healthcare facilities (25).

The impacts on health care workers during the COVID-19 pandemic highlight the need for mental health support programs. Support programs should be implemented routinely, tailored to the intensity and frequency of challenges confronting health workers. Both tangible and intangible benefits should be considered and provided for workers as needed during specific times.

This study had some limitations. The generalizability of this study is limited due to the collection of information from a small and non-representative sample. Additionally, the information reflected the experiences of a small group of workers in a few areas of health care work and in one hospital. There are two public and one private hospital in Grenada. The experience of workers may differ across the facilities. Although unlikely, recall bias may also be a limitation of this study. Statistical analysis was not conducted to determine whether there were relationships between demographic characteristics of participants and any outcomes. Further studies will be needed to identify what factors may contribute to behaviors among health workers in Grenada.

Finally, this study may serve as a pilot, providing insights into the OSH situation in clinics, laboratories and treatment centers throughout Grenada and other Caribbean countries. While other studies are awaited, the Ministry of Health and private administrators should begin planning and implementing programs to improve occupational health in health care settings. These programs can benefit from future studies to strengthen and mainstream activities to better address the needs of workers. The following are recommendations to immediately address OSH challenges at the General Hospital:

1. Develop a health and safety management system to reduce accidents, injuries, and health hazards at the hospital to evaluate work designs, staff shortages, and taking breaks between shifts.
2. Educate workers on health hazards and preventable methods when dealing with hazards.
3. Improve administrative and engineering controls to reduce workers exposure to health hazards.
4. Employ an occupational health officer to monitor, evaluate, and report to administrators on occupational health issues such as ensuring all workers are wearing their PPEs and follow OSH protocols at the hospital.
5. Provide psychological support for workers who may feel overwhelmed.
6. This study focused on four job categories at the hospital. Future studies may include other categories such as doctors, pharmacists, and other staff members.
7. Future research can explore OSH for other categories of healthcare workers at the hospital using a quantitative methodology so that generalizations can be made.
8. Conduct comparative analysis on occupational hazards at private healthcare facilities and government owned.
9. Patients' perception of safety and health hazards can also be investigated in future.
10. Future studies can investigate how the OSH concerns affect motivation and productivity of the participants.

Conclusion

In this study, participants reported being exposed to biological, psychosocial, ergonomic, and physical health hazards at the General Hospital. The biological hazards included poor handling and disposal of needles, and exposure to saliva, blood, feces, and urine. Workplace design, high uncertainty due to OSH measures, long working hours, fear of contracting infectious diseases due to limited supply of PPE and burnout were reported as psychosocial hazards.

Ergonomic and physical hazards included low level of knowledge on safe lifting and experiencing slips and bruises, respectively.

Participants reported having similar OSH challenges prior to and during COVID-19 with the emergence of other challenges. One of the main OSH challenges prior to COVID-19 was PPE shortage, however, supplies increased during the pandemic. Appropriate sizes of PPE remained a challenge during the pandemic. Low job motivation, unpredictable working hours due to staff shortage, and inadequate planning and organizing of training became more prominent during the COVID-19 pandemic.

This study may be considered as a pilot. Further studies are necessary with a larger group and segment of the health workforce from both private and public facilities. A quantitative study methodology can be employed to assess the prevalence of issues; however, qualitative methodology will provide an opportunity for details, crucial for the development of policies and interventions to remediate identified challenges.

Acknowledgments

The authors express gratitude to the administration of the Ministry of Health in Grenada. Special thanks to Dr. Carol McIntosh and the workers at the General Hospital who participated in the study.

Disclosure

The authors declare no conflict of interest.

Appendix A

Research questionnaire

Please answer all questions honestly.

1.	What gender do you identify as?	
	Male	☐
	Female	☐
	Prefer not to say	☐
	Other _ (specify)	☐
2.	What is your age range?	
	18- 25	☐
	26-35	☐
	36- 45	☐
	45-50	☐
3.	What is your highest level of qualification?	
	Bachelor's degree	☐
	High school diploma	☐
	Less than a high school diploma	☐
	Master's degree	☐
	No degree	☐
	Other (specify)	☐
4.	What is your marital status?	
	Married	☐
	Divorced	☐
	Separated	☐
	Widowed	☐
	Unmarried	☐
	Single	☐
5.	How many years have you been employed at the General Hospital?	
	5 years	☐
	5 – 10 years	☐
	10- 20 years	☐
	Over 20 years	☐
6.	What is your job title?	
	Nurse	☐
	Lab technician	☐
	Medical waste handler	☐
	Orderly	☐
7.	How satisfied are you with the current safety and occupational health measures at work?	
	Very satisfied	☐
	Satisfied	☐
	Dissatisfied	☐
	Neither satisfied nor dissatisfied	☐
	Very dissatisfied	☐
8.	Have you suffered any accidents or injuries while performing duties at the General Hospital?	
	Yes	☐
	No	☐
	If yes, what are the cause(s) of such injury/accident?	☐
	Lack of training on health and safety	☐
	Unavailability of personal protective equipment	☐
	Ignorance on health and safety	☐
	Other	☐
9.	Are you required to wear personal protective equipment while performing your duties?	
	Yes	☐
	No	☐
10.	Have you been impacted by COVID-19 pandemic while on the job?	
	Yes	☐
	No	☐

Appendix B

Interview questions

1. How safe do you feel while carrying out your work functions?
2. What workplace health hazards you are exposed to?
3. How often have you gotten a sick leave?
4. How would you describe your job motivation within the last 5 years?
5. What are some factors that influence job motivation, productivity, and performance of workers?
6. What measures are in place to address safety and health concerns of employees?
7. What are some safety protocols that exist at the at the General Hospital?
8. Do you feel sufficiently trained in safety procedures and protocols such as using personal protective equipment on the job?
9. Explain workplace safety and health hazards prior to COVID-19 pandemic
10. What are the workplace health and safety challenges that have developed due to the Covid-19 pandemic?

Probing questions

1. On a scale of 1-10, to what extent are you affected by the COVID-19 pandemic in your workplace?
2. What types of safety training did you receive to perform your role?
3. Do you feel comfortable reporting unsafe work practices and issues to your health administrator(s)?
4. Can you list some of the changes that have emerged in your workplace due to the COVID-19 pandemic?

References

[1] United States Department of Labor. Workplace safety in hospitals: Caring for our caregivers. DOL 2022 URL: https://www.osha.gov/hospitals#:~:text=In%202019%2C%20U.S.%20hospitals%20recorded,private%20industry%20as%20a%20whole.

[2] Che Huei L, Ya-Wen L, Chiu Ming Y, Li Chen H, Jong Yi W, Ming Hung, L. Occupational health and safety hazards faced by healthcare professionals in Taiwan: A systematic review of risk factors and control strategies. SAGE Open Med 2020;8 :2050312120918999.

[3] Rai R, El-Zaemey S, Dorji N, Rai BD, Fritschi L. Exposure to occupational hazards among health care workers in low- and middle-income countries: A Scoping review. Int J Environ Res Public Health 2021;18(5):2603.

[4] Subramaniam C, Shamsudin FM, Alshuaibi ASI. Investigating employees' perceptions of workplace safety and safety compliance using PLS-SEM among technical employees in Malaysia. J Appl Struct Equation Modeling 2017;1(1):44-61.

[5] Joseph B, Joseph M. The health of the healthcare workers. Indian J Occup Environ Med 2016;20(2):71-72.

[6] Duncan JP. Occupational safety and health in the Caribbean: Challenges and opportunities for achieving development goals. West Indian Med J 2021;69(6):377.

[7] Giuffrida A, Iunes RF, Savedoff WD. Economic and health effects of occupational hazards in Latin America and the Caribbean. Washington, DC: Inter-American Development Bank, 2001.

[8] Mafham MM, Spata E, Goldacre R, Gair D, Curnow P, Bray M, et al. Covid-19 pandemic and admission rates for and management of acute coronary syndromes in England. Lancet 2020;396(10248):381-9.

[9] Schwartz J, King CC, Yen MY. Protecting healthcare workers during the coronavirus disease 2019 (COVID-19) outbreak: Lessons from Taiwan's severe acute respiratory syndrome response. Clin Infect Dis 2020;71(15):858-60.

[10] Aluko OO, Adebayo AE, Adebisi TF, Ewegbemi MK, Abidoye AT, Popoola BF. Knowledge, attitudes and perceptions of occupational hazards and safety practices in Nigerian healthcare workers. BMC Res Notes 2016;6;9:7.

[11] Sabita K, Shahi M, Bharati S, Sulata K. Knowledge and preventive practice of occupational health hazards among nurses in different teaching hospitals. IJMHS 2018;8(12):225-34.

[12] O'Connor T, Flynn M, Weinstock D, Zanoni J. Occupational safety and health education and training for underserved populations. New Solut 2014;24(1):83-106.

[13] Hickam DH, Severance S, Feldstein A, Ray L, Gorman P, Schuldheis S, Hersh WR, Krages KP, Helfand M. The effect of health care working conditions on patient safety: Summary. Evid Rep Technol Assess (Summ) 2003;74:1-3.

[14] King KC, Strony R. Needlestick. StatPearls 2022.

[15] Joukar F, Mansour-Ghanaei F, Naghipour M, Asgharnezhad M. Needlestick Injuries among healthcare workers: Why they do not report their incidence? Iran J Nurs Midwifery Res 2018;23(5):382–7.

[16] Saadeh R, Khairallah K, Abozeid H, Al Rashdan L, Alfaqih M, Alkhatatbeh, O. Needle stick and sharp injuries among healthcare workers: A retrospective six-year study. Sultan Qaboos Univ Med J 2020;20(1):e54–62.

[17] Motaarefi H, Mahmoudi H, Mohammadi E, Hasanpour-Dehkordi A. Factors associated with needlestick injuries in healthcare occupations: A systematic review. J Clin Diagn Res 2016;10(8):IE01–4.

[18] Mengistu DA, Tolera ST. Prevalence of occupational exposure to needle-stick injury and associated factors among healthcare workers of developing countries: Systematic review. J Occup Health 2020;62(1):e12179.

[19] Hempel S, Xenakis L, Danz M. Systematic reviews for occupational safety and health questions: Resources for evidence synthesis. Santa Monica, CA: RAND, Report No RR-1463-CDC, 2016.

[20] Jeleff M, Traugott M, Jirovsky-Platter E, Jordakieva G, Kutalek R. Occupational challenges of healthcare workers during the Covid-19 pandemic: a qualitative study. BMJ Open 2022;12(3):e054516.

[21] Ndejjo R, Musinguzi G, Yu X, Buregyeya E, Musoke D, Wang JS, e al. Occupational health hazards among healthcare workers in Kampala, Uganda. J Environ Public Health 2015;2015:913741.

[22] Onoja-Alexander M, Zakari U, Alexander O, Umar A, Ajumoka E, Igboanusi CJC, et al. Occupational health hazards among medical waste handlers in Ahmadu Bello University Teaching Hospital Zaria Northwest Nigeria. Infect Control Hosp Epidemiol 2020;41(S1):S334.

[23] Okeafor CU, Alamina FE. A qualitative study on psychosocial hazards among health care workers in a tertiary health facility in South-South Nigeria. Ann Ib Postgrad Med 2018;16:23-9.

[24] Wagner A, Rieger MA, Manser T, Sturm H, Hardt J, Martus P, Lessing C, Hammer A. Healthcare professionals' perspectives on working conditions, leadership, and safety climate: a cross-sectional study. BMC Health Serv Res 2019;19(1):53.

[25] Franklin P, Gkiouleka A. A Scoping review of psychosocial risks to health workers during the Covid-19 pandemic. Int J Environ Res Public Health 2021;18(5):2453.

Section three: Acknowledgments

Chapter 14

About the editors

Emmanuel O Keku, MD, MA, MSPH, trained in medicine and public health epidemiology at the University of North Carolina at Chapel Hill, School of Medicine and Public Health, Chapel Hill, North Carolina, United States. His emphasis is on chronic and infectious diseases epidemiology and has extensive research experience, research grant and trophy awards. His teaching and research career are ongoing, along with other professional commitments. He was a fellow at Genetic Approaches to Complex Heart, Lung, and Blood Diseases at The Jackson Laboratory, Bar Harbor, ME, and at the 28th ten-Day Seminar on the Epidemiology and Prevention of CVD, American Heart Association, Tahoe City, CA. He was co-PI (Phase I) and co-Investigator (Phase II) of Jackson Heart Study (JHS), multi-institutional (University of Mississippi Medical school, Jackson State University, and Tugaloo College). JHS is a longitudinal study of cardiovascular diseases risk factors in African Americans of Jackson, Mississippi. The study is funded by NHLBI since 1999. Dr. Keku developed the surveillance system for JHS. He was co-PI of Excellence in partnerships for community outreach, research, on health disparities and training, "Project Export." He was the PI for the center of Excellence in Minority Health CVD core/component: Obesity Reduction through Mall-Walk in Ethnic Minority Population, Jackson, MS, funded by NIH and NCMHD. He is a Professor and the Track Director of MD/MPH (Preventive Medicine) at the Department of Public Health and Preventive Medicine, School of Medicine, St. George's University, St George, Grenada, West Indies. He mentors undergraduate, graduate and medical students. He recently directed and completed trend analysis of both breast and prostate cancer in Grenada, West Indies. His teaching and research activities are centered on chronic diseases epidemiology, infectious diseases epidemiology, community and preventive medicine. He is actively involved in several technical and governmental committees that focus on chronic and infectious diseases prevention. He serves as a peer reviewer for several national and international grant agencies, and journals. Research interests: Chronic disease epidemiology, cancer, cardiovascular diseases (CVD), obesity, nutritional determinants of chronic diseases, genetic determinants of diseases and clinical trials, but also infectious disease epidemiology, emerging infectious disease, HIV and HPV. Email: ekeku@sgu.edu

Joav Merrick, MD, MMedSci, DMSc, born and educated in Denmark is professor of pediatrics, Division of Pediatrics, Hadassah Hebrew University Medical Center, Mt Scopus Campus, Jerusalem, Israel and Kentucky Children's Hospital, University of Kentucky, Lexington, Kentucky United States and professor of public health at the Center for Healthy Development, School of Public Health, Georgia State University, Atlanta, United States, the former medical director of the Health Services, Division for Intellectual and Developmental Disabilities, Ministry of Social Affairs and Social Services, Jerusalem, the founder and director of the National Institute of Child Health and Human Development in Israel. Numerous publications in the field of pediatrics, child health and human development, rehabilitation, intellectual disability, disability, health, welfare, abuse, advocacy, quality of life and prevention. Received the Peter Sabroe Child Award for outstanding work on behalf of Danish Children in 1985 and the International LEGO-Prize ("The Children's Nobel Prize") for an extraordinary contribution towards improvement in child welfare and well-being in 1987. In 2017 appointed a Kentucky Colonel by the Commonwealth of Kentucky, the highest honor the governor can bestow to a person. Email: jmerrick@zahav.net.il

Chapter 15

About St George's University, Department of Public Health, and Preventive Medicine (SGU-DPHPM), St George's, Grenada

Department of Public Health and Preventive Medicine (SGU-DPHPM) was established in 1999 to develop and deliver its Master of Public Health (MPH) graduate program. SGU as an international center of medical education welcomed the opportunity to train medical students and graduates in public health towards strengthening primary health care and serve capacity building for the Caribbean region towards its health systems strengthening. Since 1999, SGU-DPHPM has graduated over one thousand healthcare professionals that serve in over 50 countries. The mission of SGU-DPHPM is to provide an academic focal point for interdisciplinary education, research, service and scholarship with a focus that is both globally relevant and locally applicable.

Education

SGU-DPHPM administers a Council on Education for Public Health (CEPH) MPH program with areas of concentration in global health, preventive medicine, veterinary public health, epidemiology, environmental and occupational health and health policy and administration. SGU-DPHPM also coordinates public health education for the Doctor of Medicine (MD) program as well as collaborates in veterinary public health for the Doctor of Veterinary Medicine (DVM) program. Additionally, SGU-DPHPM provides graduate course for students in the School of Graduate Studies Masters and Doctoral programs, a Certificate in Public Health program for public health practitioners and supports workforce development and community health education through ongoing training initiatives. Students and graduates of SGU-DPHPM MPH program successfully enhance their graduate public health experience with a commitment to lifelong learning as Certified Public Health (CPH) professionals from the United States National Board of Public Health Examiners (NBPHE).

Research activities

The affiliated faculty of SGU-DPHPM over the years have published work from projects and research activities thorough national and international collaborations. For the past 20 years, in collaboration with SGU's research institute, Windward Islands Research and Education Foundation (WINDREF), SGU-DPHPM faculty, students and project/research partners and collaborators have administered over 10 million USD in grant funding and over 250 publications across peer reviewed journals and national and international publications. SGU-DPHPM research is supported by SGU's Office of Research which includes access to institutional funding and support as well as Institutional Review Board (IRB) and Institutional Animal Care and Use Committee (IACUC) which serves to review research work for ethical clearance. SGU-DPHPM research is coordinated with the research institute Windward Islands Research and Education Foundation (WINDREF). WINDREF, established in 1994 is registered as a 501(c)3 in the United States, a Charitable Trust in the United Kingdom and a Non-Governmental Organization in Grenada. Through WINDREF's coordination with administrative support, laboratory capacity, grants management, statistical support and network of research fellows, SGU-DPHPM faculty and students are actively engaged in research activities.

Service

Over the past 20th years of SGU-DPHPM, many activities became focused on collaboration with various local, regional and international initiatives, which has resulted in collaboration around the establishment of a World Health Organization (WHO) Collaborating Center in Environmental and Occupational Health. Also, in response to the disproportionate and adverse effects of the climate on health, a United Nations Frame Convention on Climate Change, Regional Collaborating Center (UNFCCC-RCC). Furthermore, SGU-DPHPM has partnered with local and regional governments and community based organizations in response to disasters, vector borne disease outbreaks and overall management of non-communicable diseases. Service activities is additionally conducted with SGU-DPHPM's active Public Health Students Association (PHSA). PHSA routinely partners with medical and veterinary students to conduct community health clinics as well as health education and environmental management service based activities across Grenada. SGU-DPHPM additionally contains the Gamma Kappa chapter of Delta Omega Honors Society which is the oldest professional public health society which prides itself on community service and informs community work in response to community assessment and identified community needs.

Scholarship

SGU-DPHPM focus on inter-professional education, research and service is lead through the scholarship of its faculty and student collaborations and in partnership with international institutions and colleagues. Details of SGU-DPHPM's scholarship can be accessed from the website (sgu.edu).

Partners and collaborations

SGU-DPHPM education, research, service and scholarship is delivered in collaborations with the Schools of Medicine, Veterinary Medicine, Arts and Sciences and Graduate Studies at SGU. SGU-DPHPM also supports local organizations in Grenada with their annual work plan which includes the Grenada Public Health Association, Grenada Diabetes Association and the Grenada Cancer Society. Regionally, SGU-DPHPM supports the work of the Organization of Eastern Caribbean States (OECS), Caribbean Public Health Agency (CARPHA) and the Pan American Health Organization (PAHO). SGU-DPHPM through memberships and fellowships are also actively involved in the work of the American Public Health Association (APHA), Association of Schools and Programs in Public Health (ASPPH), Consortium on Universities in Public Health (CUGH), Royal Society of Public Health (RSPH), Royal Society of Tropical Medicine and Hygiene (RSTMH) and global agencies such as World Health Organization (WHO), World Bank and the United Nations (UN). Funding partnership and collaborations is engaged through agencies such as the National Institutes of Health (NIH), World Bank, World Diabetes Foundation (WDF), United Nations Development Program (UNDP) United Nations Global Environmental Facility (UN-GEF), Centers for Disease Control and Prevention (CDC), National Institutes for Occupational Safety and Health (NIOSH), United States Department of

Agriculture (USDA), Public Health Canada, African Medical Research and Education Foundation (AMREF) and the Caribbean Community (CARICOM) and Caribbean Public Health Agency (CARPHA). SGU-DPHPM with its interdisciplinary local to global focus have also partners with several institutions in the Caribbean; T.A. Marryshaw Community College (TAMCC), University of the West Indies, University of Trinidad and Tobago, University of Technology, Jamaica, Pasteur Institute, Guadeloupe, Institute of Tropical Medicine, Cuba, North America; New York University (NYU), State University of New York (SUNY), Sanford University, John's Hopkins University Bloomberg School of Public Health (JHU), Colombia University, Mailman School of Public Health, South America; Universidad de Antioquia, Colombia, University of Guyana, Guyana, Europe; Northumbria University (NU) and the Royal Veterinary College (RVC), UK, Swiss Tropical Medicine Institute, Switzerland, Africa; Juba Medical College, South Sudan, University of Kwa-Zulu, Natal, South Africa, Makerere University, Uganda, Asia; Mahidol University and Kasetsart University, Thailand, Chitkara University, MS Ramaiah Medical College and Indian Institute of Health Management Research (IIHMR), India, Konkuk University, South Korea and Polytechnic Institute in Singapore.

Contact

Emmanuel O Keku, MD, MA, MSPH, Professor and Track Director, MD/MPH program, School of Medicine, St George's University, Department of Public Health, and Preventive Medicine, POBox 7, St George, Grenada, West Indies.

Email: ekeku@sgu.edu.

Chapter 16

About the National Institute of Child Health and Human Development in Israel

The National Institute of Child Health and Human Development (NICHD) in Israel was established in 1998 as a virtual institute under the auspices of the Medical Director, Ministry of Social Affairs and Social Services in order to function as the research arm for the Office of the Medical Director. In 1998 the National Council for Child Health and Pediatrics, Ministry of Health and in 1999 the Director General and Deputy Director General of the Ministry of Health endorsed the establishment of the NICHD.

Mission

The mission of a National Institute for Child Health and Human Development in Israel is to provide an academic focal point for the scholarly interdisciplinary study of child life, health, public health, welfare, disability, rehabilitation, intellectual disability and related aspects of human development. This mission includes research, teaching, clinical work, information and public service activities in the field of child health and human development.

Service and academic activities

Over the years many activities became focused in the south of Israel due to collaboration with various professionals at the Faculty of Health Sciences (FOHS) at the Ben Gurion University of the Negev (BGU). Since 2000 an affiliation with the Zusman Child Development Center at the Pediatric Division of Soroka University Medical Center has resulted in collaboration around the establishment of the Down Syndrome Clinic at that center. In 2002 a full course on "Disability" was established at the Recanati School for Allied Professions in the Community, FOHS, BGU and in 2005 collaboration was started with the Primary Care Unit of the faculty and disability became part of the master of public health course on "Children and society". In the academic year 2005-2006 a one semester course on "Aging with disability" was started as part of the master of science program in gerontology in our collaboration with the Center for Multidisciplinary Research in Aging. In 2010 collaborations with the Division of Pediatrics, Hadassah Hebrew University Medical Center, Jerusalem, Israel around the National Down Syndrome Center and teaching students and residents about intellectual and developmental disabilities as part of their training at this campus.

Research activities

The affiliated staff have over the years published work from projects and research activities in this national and international collaboration. In the year 2000 the International Journal of Adolescent Medicine and Health and in 2005 the International Journal on Disability and Human Development of De Gruyter Publishing House (Berlin and New York) were affiliated with the National Institute of Child Health and Human Development. From 2008 also the International Journal of Child Health and Human Development (Nova Science, New York), the International Journal of Child and Adolescent Health (Nova Science) and the Journal of Pain Management (Nova Science) affiliated and from 2009 the International Public Health Journal (Nova Science) and Journal of Alternative Medicine Research (Nova Science). All peer-reviewed international journals.

National collaborations

Nationally the NICHD works in collaboration with the Faculty of Health Sciences, Ben Gurion University of the Negev; Department of Physical Therapy, Sackler School of Medicine, Tel Aviv University; Autism Center, Assaf HaRofeh Medical Center; National Rett and PKU Centers at Chaim Sheba Medical Center, Tel HaShomer; Department of Physiotherapy, Haifa University; Department of Education, Bar Ilan University, Ramat Gan, Faculty of Social Sciences and Health Sciences; College of Judea and Samaria in Ariel and in 2011 affiliation with Center for Pediatric Chronic Diseases and

National Center for Down Syndrome, Department of Pediatrics, Hadassah Hebrew University Medical Center, Mount Scopus Campus, Jerusalem.

International collaborations

Internationally with the Department of Disability and Human Development, College of Applied Health Sciences, University of Illinois at Chicago; Strong Center for Developmental Disabilities, Golisano Children's Hospital at Strong, University of Rochester School of Medicine and Dentistry, New York; Centre on Intellectual Disabilities, University of Albany, New York; Centre for Chronic Disease Prevention and Control, Health Canada, Ottawa; Chandler Medical Center and Children's Hospital, Kentucky Children's Hospital, Section of Adolescent Medicine, University of Kentucky, Lexington; Chronic Disease Prevention and Control Research Center, Baylor College of Medicine, Houston, Texas; Division of Neuroscience, Department of Psychiatry, Columbia University, New York; Institute for the Study of Disadvantage and Disability, Atlanta; Center for Autism and Related Disorders, Department Psychiatry, Children's Hospital Boston, Boston; Department of Pediatric and Adolescent Medicine, Western Michigan University Homer Stryker MD School of Medicine, Kalamazoo, Michigan, United States; Department of Paediatrics, Child Health and Adolescent Medicine, Children's Hospital at Westmead, Westmead, Australia; International Centre for the Study of Occupational and Mental Health, Düsseldorf, Germany; Centre for Advanced Studies in Nursing, Department of General Practice and Primary Care, University of Aberdeen, Aberdeen, United Kingdom; Quality of Life Research Center, Copenhagen, Denmark; Nordic School of Public Health, Gottenburg, Sweden, Scandinavian Institute of Quality of Working Life, Oslo, Norway; The Department of Applied Social Sciences (APSS) of The Hong Kong Polytechnic University Hong Kong.

Targets

Our focus is on research, international collaborations, clinical work, teaching and policy in health, disability and human development and to establish the NICHD as a permanent institute in Israel in order to conduct model research and policy.

Contact

Professor Joav Merrick, MD, MMedSci, DMSc
Director, National Institute of Child Health and Human Development, Jerusalem, Israel.
Email: jmerrick@zahav.net.il.

Section four: Index

Index

A

B

C

T

U

W

Y